The Nursing Process

Commissioning Editor: Susan Young
Development Editor: Catherine Jackson
Project Manager: David Fleming
Designer: Stewart Larking
Illustration Manager: Bruce Hogarth

The Nursing Process: A Global Concept

Edited by

Monika Habermann DrPhil RN

Professor of Nursing; Head of the Centre of Nursing Research and Counselling; Head of the International Study Course of Nursing Management, Zentrum für Pflegeforschung und Beratung, Hochschule Bremen, Germany

Leana R. Uys D Soc Sc (Nursing) RN RM

Deputy Vice Chancellor; Head of College of Health Sciences, University of KwaZulu-Natal, Durban, South Africa

With a foreword by

Barbara Parfitt PhD RGN RNM

Dean of the School of Nursing, Midwifery and Community Health, Glasgow Caledonian University, Glasgow, UK

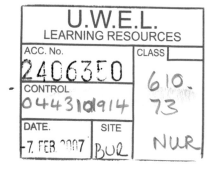
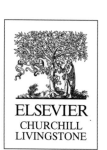

ELSEVIER
CHURCHILL
LIVINGSTONE

EDINBURGH LONDON NEW YORK OXFORD PHILADELPHIA ST LOUIS SYDNEY TORONTO 2006

ELSEVIER
CHURCHILL
LIVINGSTONE

First published 2005

ISBN 0 443 10191 4

British Library Cataloguing in Publication Data
A catalogue record for this book is available from the British Library

Library of Congress Cataloging in Publication Data
A catalog record for this book is available from the Library of Congress

Notice
Knowledge and best practice in this field are constantly changing. As new research
and experience broaden our knowledge, changes in practice, treatment and drug
therapy may become necessary or appropriate. Readers are advised to check the
most current information provided (i) on procedures featured or (ii) by the
manufacturer of each product to be administered, to verify the recommended dose
or formula, the method and duration of administration, and contraindications.
It is the responsibility of the practitioner, relying on their own experience and
knowledge of the patient, to make diagnoses, to determine dosages and the best
treatment for each individual patient, and to take all appropriate safety
precautions. To the fullest extent of the law, neither the publisher nor the editors
assumes any liability for any injury and/or damage.

The Publisher

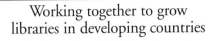

Working together to grow
libraries in developing countries

www.elsevier.com | www.bookaid.org | www.sabre.org

ELSEVIER   BOOK AID
             International   Sabre Foundation

your source for books,
journals and multimedia
in the health sciences

www.elsevierhealth.com

The
publisher's
policy is to use
**paper manufactured
from sustainable forests**

Printed in China

Contents

Contributors

Elske Ammenwerth PhD
*Associate Professor of Health Informatics, UMIT
(University for Health Sciences, Medical Informatics
and Technology), Hall, Tyrol, Austria*

Barbara Stevens Barnum RN, PhD, FAAN
*Professor, Retired, Columbia University New York,
USA*

Niels Buus MN RN
*PhD student, University of Southern Denmark,
Denmark and the Centre for Innovation in Nursing
Education, Aarhus, Denmark*

Chris Game RN RM DipNEd MEdStud
*Secretary, New South Wales Division, National
Tertiary Education Union, Sydney, New South
Wales, Australia*

Monika Habermann DrPhil RN
*Professor of Nursing; Head of the Centre of Nursing
Research and Counselling; Head of the International
Study Course of Nursing Management, Zentrum für
Pflegeforschung und Beratung, Hochschule Bremen,
Germany*

Hermi Hewitt PhD RN RM
*Head and Senior Lecturer, The UWI School of
Nursing, Mona, University of the West Indies, Mona
Campus, Kingston, Jamaica*

Marja Kaunonen PhD RN
*Senior Assistant Professor, Department of Nursing
Science, University of Tampere, Tampere, Finland*

Daniel Kelly PhD MSc BSc RN PGCE
*Senior Research Fellow, St Bartholomew School of
Nursing, City University, London, UK*

Alena Mellanová PhD EdD RN
*Senior Lecturer, Institute of Nursing Theory and
Practice, 1st Faculty of Medicine, Charles University,
Prague, Czech Republic*

Barbara Parfitt PhD RGN RNM
*Dean of the School of Nursing, Midwifery and
Community Health, Glasgow Caledonian University,
Glasgow, UK*

Bev Taylor PhD MEd RN RM
*Foundation Chair in Nursing, School of Nursing and
Health Care Practices, Southern Cross University,
New South Wales, Australia*

Michael Traynor PhD MA RN HV
*Professor of Nursing, School of Health and Social
Sciences, Middlesex University, London, UK*

Leana R. Uys D Soc Sc (Nursing) RN RM
*Deputy Vice Chancellor; Head of College of Health
Sciences, University of KwaZulu-Natal, Durban,
South Africa*

Maritta Välimäki PhD RN
*Senior Assistant Professor, Department of
Nursing Science, University of Tampere, Tampere,
Finland*

Martin F. Ward MPhil RMN DipNurs RNT
CertEd NEBSS Dip
*Independent Mental Health Nursing Consultant;
Coordinator of Mental Health, University of Malta,
Malta*

Foreword

Barbara Parfitt

In the 1980s, when I returned from working overseas to Britain, I discovered the phenomena of the Nursing Process. I was asked to assist with its introduction into practice in the district hospital. It was a challenging and difficult task that met with considerable resistance. The great mistake that was made at that time in Britain was to focus on the paperwork associated with its introduction rather than the thought process that it promoted. Nurses were resistant to what they perceived as the massive increase in workload with the added burden of having to complete complicated records using terms of which they were unsure. Carrying out nursing assessments and distinguishing nursing objectives from medical tasks was a major challenge and seemed far removed from the delivery of care.

These were the early days, and I realized at that time that, if it were to be fully understood, the Nursing Process had to be recognized and experienced as a thought process and not a paper exercise. In order to help the nurses understand the concept of the Nursing Process, I threw away the paperwork and tried to introduce the logical systematic thinking pathway that the process identified.

Nurses soon grasped the notion of systematic scientific thinking, and recognized how the process enabled them to undertake a logical analysis of a clinical situation and make the required decisions. They learned how to implement care in a systematic way and, more importantly, how to evaluate its effectiveness. Use of the process in

reality was a major driver that moved nurses away from task-orientated care to a holistic approach. It allowed for the expression of different nursing theories demonstrating how priorities change according to the underpinning philosophy of care being used and provided the groundwork for the development of evidence-based practice. Scholarly and critical approaches to care were reinforced and a mechanism was provided for the development of an objective evaluation and review of practice. The introduction of this scientific thinking into nursing has changed the way that nurses think and work.

The amazing thing about the process is that it is culturally and professionally neutral. It is a tool that can be understood and applied in every country, as it provides an accessible means to support evidence-based practice that is contextual. The process itself is a means to an end and is not exclusive to nursing. It can be applied in many situations, and nurses, once they have understood the basic concept and thought process, are able to use the process to transfer this skill into other situations. It thus becomes a means of empowerment.

This book provides a unique opportunity for readers to explore in a critical fashion the spread of the use of the process over the last 25 years. It is the first book of its kind that examines the impact of the Nursing Process on the profession within an international context. The book highlights the history of the process and examines its contribution to decision-making, management of care and research. It reviews the way in which the process has been or is used within a number of different countries.

The process is now an integral part of nursing practice worldwide, and is recognized and acknowledged by nurses everywhere. Its global acceptance is a key indicator of the professional status of the nurse and the scientific nature of our discipline.

The content of this book is both stimulating and challenging. It will provide a useful text for postgraduate students, academics and those who are interested in the utilization of nursing research and the history of change within the profession.

Acknowledgement

We thank Rosemary Cadman for her valuable language editing and advice.

Chapter 1

The Nursing Process: globalization of a nursing concept – an introduction

Leana Uys and Monika Habermann

THE NURSING PROCESS – A KEY CONCEPT OF NURSING

The concept of the Nursing Process was developed in the USA in the 1960s and became associated with the books published by Yura and Walsh (1967, 1978, 1983). Since then, the Nursing Process has been regarded as the key element of advanced, theoretically based nursing practice, bringing into reality what Yura and Walsh stated in one of their introductions: 'The Nursing Process is the core and essence of nursing: it is central to all nursing actions; it is applicable in any setting . . . (it) provide(s) a base from which all systematic actions can proceed' (1983: 1). Global organizations, such as the World Health Organization (WHO) and the International Council for Nurses (ICN) validated this evaluation by using the Nursing Process as a central concept, while national governments and nursing organizations based their legal prescription of quality nursing on the Nursing Process, for example, Sweden, Germany, UK, South Africa, State Practice Acts in the USA, the American Nursing Association (ANA) and the United Kingdom Central Council for Nursing, Midwifery and Health Visitors (UKCC). Countries in which nursing had developed outside the Anglo-Saxon sphere of influence up to the end of the 20th century, such as the Czech Republic, recently followed this trend (see Mellanová, Chapter 11 in this volume). The Nursing Process thus represents a global concept that is being taught, discussed and implemented worldwide.

The Nursing Process is grounded in a problem-solving cycle, which usually includes at least the following phases:

- collecting information and assessing the patient;
- planning the care and defining the relevant objectives for nursing care;
- implementing actual interventions; and
- evaluating the results.

In some regions, a cycle of five or six phases is used by further differentiating steps, possibly to guide the planning and actual nurses' actions in even more detail. Such additional steps may cover, for instance, 'making a diagnosis', 'setting objectives' and 'planning' or 'collecting information', and 'defining problems and resources' – see Välimäki and Kaunonen (Chapter 6), Taylor and Game (Chapter 8), and Uys (Chapter 9) in this volume.

Theories of nursing and the respective instruments of assessment that underlie the process vary within and between countries. There does seem to be a consensus that the Nursing Process should be based on patient-centred care, which requires the involvement of the patient and relevant others in all the phases of the process.

The structure of the Nursing Process and the underlying nursing theories that are used are supposed to guide the production of nursing care plans and the documentation of care in all fields of nursing. The nursing care plan is, therefore, the concrete form which makes explicit the process orientation in nursing. As such, it is supposed to enhance systematic care and to operate additionally as a vehicle for communication, fostering continuity and visibility of care (Mason 1999: 380). Many practitioners and researchers view the concept of the Nursing Process and the instrument to set it into action (the care plan) as interwoven in such a way as to represent two sides of the same coin. Research about care plans, therefore, documents the state of art of the Nursing Process and vice versa.

IMPLEMENTATION AND EVALUATION OF THE NURSING PROCESS

Despite the international perception of the Nursing Process as the core concept of nursing and its legal standing in many countries, there are a number of problems with regard to the process. Firstly, the Nursing Process is still only partially implemented in practice in most countries, although it is now 40 years since its introduction. The reasons for this limited implementation are manifold. To understand these, we have to look at the history of nursing, as exemplified in some chapters of this book. We also need to analyse the construction of good quality nursing and the ambiguous – in effect, often contradictory – national and international legal and financial contexts in which care is provided by nurses (Finland, Australia). Finally, we have to understand the development and dimensions of theorizing in nursing, the unfolding of an ongoing discourse searching for meaning and power in national and international health policies. Some exploratory outlines considering these dimensions will be given in the following sections.

Research results and professional reports stress the fact that the Nursing Process is not well accepted by the practitioners who have to put the system into practice. These problems with implementation have been described in a series of studies. Sharitts (1988) showed in a study undertaken in nine metropolitan hospitals in the USA that the act and quality of implementation decreased with each succeeding step. Several studies in diverse countries have indicated that the formulation of adequate objectives and the evaluation of the outcomes are often not included in the process (Morissay-Ross 1988, in Mason 1999, Howse and Bailey 1992, Krohwinkel 1993, Höhmann et al 1996, 1997, 1998, Mason 1999, Güttler and Lehmann 2003; see also individual country reports in this volume). O'Connel's grounded theory study (1998) on implementation pointed to several problems with the clinical application of the Nursing Process. A chart review carried out by Murphy et al (2000) in psychiatric units showed a very low level of implementation of all steps. For instance, in only 6–7% of records were problems identified based on the assessment that was performed, and in only 12% were problems explicitly stated. Krohwinkel (1993) found in an intervention study that incomplete implementation of the Nursing Process, including insufficient documentation, contributed to poor outcomes of the nursing care for stroke patients. She also found, as others (Höhmann 1998, Mason 1999, Güttler and Lehmann 2003), that the elaboration of the care plan was rarely realized with the patient or relevant others. The plan was checked and written at the end of the shift and not attended to when starting the shift, so that it did not guide the actual work.

In addition to the problems concerning the fragmented implementation of the total process cycle, nursing care plans had been found to be illegible, confusing, lacking actuality, validity and reliability (Krohwinkel 1993, Höhmann et al 1996, 1997, Güttler and Lehmann 2003). Even if plans are available in a formally correct form, nursing care plans are still often handled by nurses as fulfilling a legal or managerial-imposed obligation (Höhmann et al 1998, Mason 1999, Güttler and Lehmann 2003). For many practitioners, working with a comprehensive Nursing Process record means getting lost in paperwork instead of dedicating available time to direct nursing care (Höhmann et al 1998, Mason 1999, Güttler and Lehmann 2003). Mason and Attree (1997) conclude that this widely observed poor acceptance of working with care plans and the imminent process-orientation shows a theory–practice gap.

The reasons put forward by many authors for the lack of implementation were widespread poor education of nurses in general, with the result that many have problems writing detailed and precise reports, formulating objectives or documenting the ongoing evaluation of care. Poor preparation for the process orientation and writing of care plans have also been blamed, as well as 'bottom-down' management strategies for implementation, the time-consuming nature of following up the process, and the undifferentiated application to all fields of nursing, whilst it was experienced as unsuitable for areas such as psychiatric nursing or intensive care units (Höhmann et al 1997, 1998, O'Connel 1998, Mason 1999, Murphy et al 2000). The ongoing reluctance of many nurses to incorporate the Nursing Process into their daily work denies its practical significance.

A final problem with the Nursing Process is the lack of evidence of its relevance for patient outcomes. Moloney and Maggs (1999), in their review of outcome studies of the Nursing Process, confirmed the previous findings of Mason and Attree (1997) and Varcoe (1997) that there is a remarkable paucity of research concerning the Nursing Process as a supposed key variable in nursing outcomes. They could find no articles that adhered to criteria for valid outcome studies. Although the authors admit that the subject might not be open to randomized control studies, in their opinion this paucity indicates insufficient development of national and international nursing research, leaving a central theory untested. Nevertheless, as an outcome of their review, they presented in some detail three studies which at least approximated to the required methodological strength. These studies provide some evidence that the Nursing Process made no difference to patient outcomes.

Even though tentative, these findings are alarming, if the substantial costs involved in working on a daily basis with detailed care plans are taken into account. Mason (1999) calculated the annual costs for different wards and pointed out that the enforced application of such a costly system should be questioned in the face of the lack of evidence to support its use.

Theoretical and professional considerations add to the critical evaluation of the significance of the concept in the practical field. In 1996, Varcoe published a very thorough analysis of such criticisms of the Nursing Process. Theoretical criticisms mainly addressed the positivistic character of the Nursing Process, which was seen as fostering linear thinking, based on a methodology oriented in natural science and seeming to exclude holistic approaches in nursing rooted in humanities. As a consequence, the person in need of care will be seen as fragmented and 'problem-laden'. Care is then aimed at 'solutions' – a terminology that implies a technological approach instead of enhancing the use of a reconstructive, hermeneutical approach and the construction of interactive intervention strategies (see also Lindsey and Hartrick 1996). Creativity may be stifled as Benner (1984) and Henderson (1987) argued, intuitive knowledge depreciated, patients muted and acted upon instead of with. Nursing experts especially would, therefore, not follow such linear constructed guidelines but use experience and intuition (Field, in Mason and Attree 1997: 1074). The evaluation of the poor implementation results disregards these considerations. Nurses are blamed as resistant to innovations, irrespective of such concepts as autonomy and expert knowledge in nursing (Fischbach 2001).

Professional criticism deals with the contention that the process was developed for nurses, to distinguish the nursing field from medicine, and not to improve care. The process was also developed theoretically and not derived from practice, and was inadequately developed and implemented. Much of the criticism is related to equating the process with the nursing diagnosis movement and with a cumbersome documentation system. Thus Varcoe (1996) came to some conclusions in her analysis regarding further contributions examining the Nursing Process. In her opinion it is necessary to clarify the concept and give explicit definitions, which may involve the distinction of psychological, social and work processes. Furthermore, there must be clarification of whether the Nursing Process is regarded as a prescription of what should be done or a description of the structuring of actual nursing work. The basic objectives in implementing or teaching the Nursing Process should also be established (e.g. improving the documentation, improving quality care, getting systematic work schemes into action, etc.).

Lindsey and Hartrick (1996) took another stance. They identified opposing characteristics underlying the established Nursing Process and new paradigms in fields of nursing, like health promotion in nursing practice. They proposed that these developments would demand that the expert nurse change role conceptions towards a facilitating, resource-oriented role and empowering strategies with clients, who are experts in their own situations, as partner. The recognition of 'patterns and themes' will replace the process-based 'problem identification'. As a result, the necessary paradigm shift to human sciences will rule out the Nursing Process.

An issue that is closely linked to the Nursing Process is the ongoing development of classification systems for nursing assessment and documentation over the last two decades. In 1992, the Omaha System was published by the Omaha Visiting Nurses Association, which is seen as very useful in outpatient settings. The North American Nursing Diagnosis Association (NANDA) published its List of Approved Diagnoses in 1994, based on a long period of research. The Home Health Care Classification, developed by Georgetown University in 1992, is very similar to the NANDA system. The International Council for Nurses (ICN) developed the International Classification for Nursing Practice of which the Beta 2 version was published in 2001. Several more international and national classification systems can be listed, such as the Nursing Intervention Classification (NIC; McCloskey and Bulechek 2002), the Nursing Outcome Classification (NOC; Johnson 2000), the Resident Assessment Instrument (RAI, Garms-Homolova 2002) used in geriatric care, or an instrument to register actions of care

(Leistungserfassung in der Pflege; LEP, Bruggen 2002), which was developed in Switzerland. In view of the growing necessity to render nursing care that is transparent and verifiable in terms of costs and quality, these classifications, so hotly debated (Powers 1999), are seen as indispensable. Especially if they can be incorporated into new software-based systems, these classifications will certainly have an impact on the debate around and implementation of the Nursing Process (Chambers 1998, Higuchi et al 1999; also Ammenwerth, this volume). This development will probably not reach all fields of nursing in the foreseeable future and it will certainly not be of relevance for many countries, owing to the costs of establishing such systems.

INNOVATION PROCESSES AND GLOBALIZATION – DISSEMINATION OF THE NURSING PROCESS

It is amazing to follow the spread of the concept of the Nursing Process. According to Yura and Walsh (1983: 21), it took only 5 years after the publishing of the first book to implement the Nursing Process as the core concept of nursing in important nursing textbooks and training manuals. Roughly 25 years later, the concept has been transported over the whole world, occupying generations of nurses on all levels and in all fields in trying to implement it. It has also been adopted by important global organizations. 'Blind spots' on the international map with regard to the Nursing Process are quick to adopt the process once they join the global nursing discourse, as happened with the fall of the Iron Curtain. For those who appraise the concept as evidence of good quality in nursing work, this is a success story. It reads differently when taking the critical theoretical and professional evaluation in many countries into account. What makes it possible that ideas and concepts, which are not yet evidence-based and have a history of doubtful utilization in the practice field, are nevertheless disseminated globally? On what structure and processes are innovations in nursing based, and how do they evolve into practice? Some, necessarily tentative, considerations will be provided in the next sections about general and nursing-related theories, the dissemination of innovations, and the embeddedness of innovations in health care global markets and the power relations within these networks.

Although many authors in the field of innovation research agree that there is no single model that explains the adoption of all innovation (Estabrook 1999: 58) Rogers' (1983) model of diffusion of innovation is one of the best known in nursing. He described a process of accepting innovations as consisting of the following steps:

- learning about the innovation (knowledge);
- becoming interested (persuasion);
- making a decision to implement it (decision);
- testing it (implementation); and,
- finally, accepting it permanently (confirmation).

In his research in the agricultural sector, Rogers found that most people took between 2.2 and 2.7 years from the time they became aware of a new innovation until they accepted it. Cavanagh and Tross (1996: 1086) point out that Rogers' model pays little attention to evaluation of change in the light of ongoing knowledge acquisition. A further criticism of Rogers' model is that it does not focus on the context in which innovation takes place. Who is presenting new ideas with credibility and what are the incentives for the individuals to test them? Innovation in this light seems to be a somewhat lonely, decontextualized business involving neutral 'testers' of sociocultural and, in terms of power relations, 'neutral' innovations.

It can be thus concluded that, although there seem to be individual factors influencing the implementation of an innovation, it would seem that international acceptance of the Nursing Process cannot be explained by such factors. Therefore, one has to look at organizational factors and the attributes of the innovation itself for the answer. In this case, organizational factors can be applied to the nursing profession within a country as well as to the single institutional setting that sets the plan into action. Both build up the relevant framework from which the innovation is launched. As has been reported above, the success of the implementation had been dependent on giving incentives such as 'progression of the profession' or using plain legal enforcement.

In addition to the individual and organizational characteristics that influence the handling of innovations, Rogers (1983) constructed a classification of social systems as either having traditional or modern norms and values, and he postulated that innovation was easier in a system with modern norms. This consideration might further assist in understanding the utilization of the Nursing Process. Modern systems, in his opinion, were characterized by: developed technology with complex occupational differentiation; an acute appreciation of science, education and training; cosmopolitan social relationships in an atmosphere where new ideas entered the system freely; and careful planning, based on economic arguments. He contrasted this with a traditional system in which technology, education and training were at a low level; communication was mainly from person to person, and within the system, rather than through mass media and with outsiders; and decisions were often not based on clear reasoning, but on group considerations.

With regard to the characteristics of innovations, Rogers (1995) proposed that the following attributes influenced their adoption: complexity, relative advantage, compatibility, triability and observability. Other authors mentioned other organizational factors, such as centralization, the presence of a champion and supporting policy (Estabrook 1999). However, this application of theoretical considerations on innovation to the spreading of the Nursing Process as central concept seems doubtful. There is, for example, no evidence that nurses of 'modern' countries are more inclined to adopt the concept than nurses rooted in a country that is classified as 'traditional'. An early review on the reception of the concept across a number of countries instead showed that the presence in 'modern' countries was based on forms of forced implementation (Needham 1990). Furthermore, dualistic conceptions of modern versus traditional settings seem too simplistic for understanding the contexts and processes, similarities and anachronisms of regional realities in a global world.

Another branch of the literature on innovation in nursing concentrates on research utilization. In 1995, one edition of the *Nursing Clinics of North America* was dedicated to the topic of research utilization. Scales have been developed to measure barriers to the implementation of research findings (Funk et al 1991) and models developed to promote research utilization (Estabrook 1999). Much of this information might also apply to the implementation of the Nursing Process. Estabrook (1999) suggests that many questions and debates around this topic still need to take place. She points out that we have too few historical studies addressing the process of innovation in nursing, we have not debated the relationship between research utilization and evidence-based practice, and that the methodology of studying research utilization is underdeveloped. As discussed above, the lack of information about research utilization indicates again that international and national nursing research has not yet been developed in such a way that at least central theories are tested.

In addition to the arguments outlined so far, comprehension of the widespread dissemination of an innovation such as the Nursing Process is deepened in the light of the globalization debate. Globalization is a multidimensional process encompassing economic, social, cultural, political and technological components (Woodward et al 1999: 3). Tickly (2001) states that 'for some, globalization is a new form of global culture, governance and civil society, which is a reality beyond the control of individual nation states'. He calls this a hyperglobalist perspective. He contrasts this perspective with that of the sceptics, who see globalization as an evil political and economic entity, which is engineered by the strong to exploit the weak, and which increases the gap between the 'haves' and the 'have nots'.

Whichever view one supports, Gwele (2003) pointed out that globalization has led to health services being seen as a trade of international proportions, consisting of people and technology moving across borders on a massive scale. These movements are backed, for instance, by the General Agreement of Trade in Services (GATS), administered by the World Trade Organization (WTO 1994), which deals specifically with trade in health services. GATS includes examples such as telemedicine and telenursing, international movement of nursing students, teachers and nursing personnel, health care tourists (people visiting a foreign country for health care), and the establishment by one country of hospitals and other facilities in another country. Such 'trade' is facilitated by regional agreements on professional licensing, such as the European Union guidelines.

One of the consequences is the migration of nurses. The WHO indicated that professional nurses are the most willing group of migrating workers worldwide, following job and income opportunities not available in the home region (WHO 1996). This migration is certainly facilitated by the creation of a global nursing culture, as established with the process orientation as a central concept, and following this in the last decade, the nursing diagnoses. Even when one does not agree with complaints like the 'poaching of nurses' from developing countries as brought up recently (e.g. Singh et al 2003: 666), global concepts give rise to scepticism. Do they indicate a global culture, representing the end of real or mentally confirmed national frontiers and an upcoming global consciousness of nurses as world citizens and a true international professional (Welsch 1999)? Or, since the evidence of positive outcomes from the Nursing Process is limited, one can speculate that the global dissemination of the Nursing Process is due to a powerful discourse led and dominated by some regions, fostered by global institutions and transported globally because they are backed by global trade approaches. In concluding this argument about focusing on the development of professional nursing, we must consider whether the concept of the Nursing Process has contributed to a professional development internationally, and what can be learnt from the dissemination and internationalization of the nursing concept.

CONCLUSION AND INTRODUCTION OF AUTHORS

The introductory literature review can be summarized as follows. The Nursing Process appears to form part of the description of quality nursing care in the legal regulations for many countries, and is included in the definition of nursing in such influential organizations as the WHO and ICN. It is a global concept and, as a result, the education of nurses internationally is based primarily on the Nursing Process, although there appears to be no evidence so far that the Nursing Process makes a difference in terms of enhancing the quality of care. Problems of implementation of the concept in practice are reported but again the nature of these problems is not clear. The concept of the Nursing Process can, therefore, be seen as deeply rooted in collective professional knowledge, guiding practice evaluations and taking steps towards quality development. New developments, such as classification systems in nursing, build on this and information technology promises new solutions to the old problem of lacking implementation. Acknowledging this, the authors of this volume have focused on illuminating national and international developments and providing debates around the concept, and have extended the discussion of several aspects.

The first section in the volume is dedicated to theoretical considerations and empirical findings. The historical and current debates concerning the Nursing Process are explored in more detail by Daniel Kelly, followed by an in-depth discourse analysis focusing on the power relations by Niels Buus and Michael Traynor. Martin Ward then looks at the implementation of the Nursing Process in mental health nursing in the UK, considering how changes in this field of care delivery have influenced implementation. In some of the reports for individual countries, the implementation of the Nursing Process in different fields of nursing is also explored, but is considered only briefly (Uys, Taylor and Game). Elske Ammerfeld's contribution analyses research outcomes with regard to the perception and use of the Nursing Process in the light of new software developments.

In-depth reports for individual countries then sum up the state of the art of nursing, drawing on all available information. Maritta Välimäki and Marja Kaunonen, two Finnish authors, represent European developments and influences in their report, since academic and practice developments in this region have similar traits. In exploring the decisive frameworks of the concept implementation in Australia, Beverly Taylor and Chris Game identify interprofessional problems as one of the major triggers that promoted the Nursing Process, even though a near total lack of national nursing research to clarify processes and outcomes was found. Development and issues in Germany exemplify the arbitrary function of the Nursing Process for professionalization. It seems that its implementation and legal embeddedness fitted well there with a concept of the nurse as a medical assistant.

The contributions of Leana Uys, Hermi Hewitt and Alena Mellanová provide evidence from the so-called 'developing countries', each representing different regions in the world. Uys details historical developments, discourses and practice implications for South Africa. She points to the poor practice impact, which is based on feelings of inadequacy owing to difficult working conditions and the severe health problems of the population. She questions how nursing plans can be developed when the rendering of basic care and therapeutic interventions are hardly realized owing to an overload of work. Hermi Hewith describes a similar stance in her report from Jamaica. The Nursing Process and the documentation involved appear to be regarded as part of a problematic colonial heritage as well as an impulse for quality development. Alena Mellanová represents one of the countries that have participated only recently in international nursing discourses. The country's adaptation to European nursing systems clearly supports nurses who occupy professional territories that have so far been dominated by medical doctors. The process of adoption in some countries implies also that international concepts and strategies are implemented without further debate. The globalization continues.

The initial question that prompted the collection of these contributions – 'The Nursing Process: core of nursing?' – will necessarily find only a tentative answer in a conclusion by Barbara Barnum, based on all the preceding chapters as well as providing deep insights into the last two decades of the development in nursing theory and practice. Within this background, Barbara Barnum also represents the USA, the country in which the concept originated.

REFERENCES

Benner P 1984 From novice to expert. Addison-Wesley, California

Bruggen v d H 2002 Pflegeklassifikationen. Huber, Bern

Cavanagh S J, Tross G 1996 Utilizing research findings in nursing: policy and practice considerations. Journal of Advanced Nursing 24: 1083–1088

Chambers S 1988 Nursing diagnosis in learning disabilities nursing. British Journal of Nursing 7(19): 1177–1181

Estabrook C A 1999 Mapping the research utilization field in nursing. Canadian Journal of Nursing Research 31(1): 53–72

Fischbach A 2001 Pflegeprozess in Diskussion. Die Schwester/Der Pfleger 40(2): 173–175

Funk S G, Champagne M T, Wiese R A, Tornquist E M 1991 Barriers: the barriers to research utilization scale. Applied Nursing Research 4(2): 90–95

Garms-Homolova V (ed.) 2002 Assessment für die häusliche Pflege. Resident Assessment Instrument – home care (RAI HC 2.0). Huber, Bern

Güttler K, Lehmann A 2003 Eine Typologie für Pflegeprozesse am Beispiel des Projektes Pflegeprozess, Standardisierung und Qualität im Dienstleistungssektor Pflege. Pflege 16: 153–160

Gwele N S 2003 Globalization and the nursing workforce: the importance of what we care about. Inaugural lecture delivered at the University of Natal, Durban

Henderson V 1987 Nursing process – a critique. Holistic Nursing Practice 1(3): 7–16

Higuchi K A, Dulberg C, Duff V 1999 Factors associated with nursing diagnosis utilisation in Canada. Nursing Diagnosis 10(4): 137–147

Höhmann U, Weinrich H, Gätschenberger G 1996 Die Bedeutung des Pflegeplanes für die Qualitätssicherung in der Pflege. Abschlussbericht Bundesministerium für Arbeit und Sozialordnung, Bonn

Höhmann U, Weinrich H, Gätschenberger G 1997 Neues Dokumentationssystem zur vereinfachten patientenbezogenen Umsetzung des Pflegeprozesses in ambulanter und stationärer Langzeitpflege. Pflege 10: 157–163

Höhmann U, Müller-Mundt G, Schulz B 1998 Qualität durch Kooperation. Gesundheitsdienste in der Vernetzung. Mabuse, Frankfurt

Howse E, Bailey I 1992 Resistance to documentation – a nursing research issue. International Journal of Nursing Studies 29(4): 371–380

Johnson M (ed.) 2000 Nursing outcome classification (NOC), 2nd edn. Mosby, New York

Krohwinkel M 1993 Der Pflegeprozess am Beispiel von Apoplexiekranken – Eine Studie zur Erfahrung und Entwicklung von Pflegeprozessqualität. Schriftenreihe des Bundesministeriums für Gesundheit, Bd. 16, Bonn

Lindsey E, Hartrick G 1996 Health-promoting nursing practice: the demise of the nursing process? Journal of Advanced Nursing 23: 106–112

Mason C 1999 Guide to practice or 'load of rubbish'? The influence of care plans on Nursing practice in five clinical areas in Northern Ireland. Journal of Advanced Nursing 29(2): 380–387

Mason G M C, Attree M 1997 The relationship between research and the nursing process in clinical practice. Journal of Advanced Nursing 26: 1045–1049

McClosky J C, Bulechek G M 2002 Nursing intervention classification (NIC). In: Oud N (ed.) ACENDIO. Huber, Bern: 31–44

Moloney R, Maggs C 1999 A systematic review of the relationships between written manual Nursing care planning, record keeping and patient outcomes. Journal of Advanced Nursing 30 (1): 51–57

Morissay-Ross M 1988 Documentation: If you haven't written it, you haven't done it. Nursing Clinics of North America 23(2): 363–372

Murphy K, Cooney A, Casey D, Connor M, Dineen B 2000 The Roper, Logan and Tierney 1996 Model: perceptions and operationalization of the model in psychiatric nursing within a Health Board in Ireland. Journal of Advanced Nursing 31(6): 1333–1341

Needham I 1990 Ansichten und Meinungen zum Pflegeprozess: Eine hermeneutische Untersuchung von Aussagen in Fachschriftenartikeln. Pflege 3(1): 59–67

O'Connel B 1998 The clinical application of the Nursing Process in selected acute care settings: a professional mirage. Australian Journal of Advanced Nursing 15(4): 22–32

Powers P 1999 Der Diskurs der Pflegediagnosen. Huber, Bern

Rogers E M 1995 Diffusion of innovations, 4th edn. New York: The Free Press

Sharrits L 1998 Investigation of the use of Nursing Process in a metropolitan area. http://www.stti.iupui.edu/rnr/search/hts/fullview.hts 22 May 2002

Singh J A, Nkala B, Amuah E, Mehta N, Ahmad A 2003 The ethics of nurses poaching from the developing world. Nursing Ethics 10(6): 666–670

Tikly L 2001 Globalization and education in the post colonial world: towards a conceptual framework. Comparative Education 37(2): 151–171

Varcoe C 1996 Disparagement of the Nursing Process: the new dogma? Journal of Advanced Nursing 23: 120–125

Welsch W 1999 Transkulturalität. Zwischen Globalisierung und Partikularisierung. In: Interkulturalität Grundprobleme der Kulturbegegnung. Mainzer Universitätsgespräche 45–72

Woodward D, Drager N, Beaglehole R, Lipson D 1999 Trade in health services: Global, regional and country perspectives. PAHO, Washington, DC

World Health Organisation 1996 Nursing practice. Report of a WHO Expert Committtee. Technical Report Series, Bd. 860. WHO, Geneva

World Trade Organization 1994 General agreement on trade in services. WTO, Geneva

Yura H, Walsh M B (eds) 1967 The nursing process. Appleton-Century-Crofts, Washington, DC

Yura H, Walsh M 1978 The nursing process: assessment, planning, implementation and evaluation, 3rd edn. Appleton-Century-Crofts, New York

Yura H, Walsh M B 1983 The nursing process: assessment, planning, implementing, evaluating. Appleton Century-Crofts, Norwalk

Chapter **2**

Opening new discourses in nursing: the history of the Nursing Process in the UK

Daniel Kelly

INTRODUCTION

The focus of this chapter is the historical development and legacy of the Nursing Process within the British National Health Service (NHS). It will be argued that the Nursing Process, originally a tool to manage care that was imported from the USA, led to a number of related developments in nursing theory and practice. The underlying philosophy of individualized patient care differed markedly from early approaches to nursing, which focused on the mastery of tasks and left decision-making to others – usually doctors. It will be argued that the Nursing Process contributed to subsequent developments in British nursing, such as the autonomy of advanced roles as well as research and theory development.

Fundamentally, the Nursing Process was based on the assessment of clinical need and the evaluation of care outcomes. Field, a Canadian nurse academic, describes the link between cognitive processes of the individual practitioner and the philosophy underpinning the Nursing Process:

> To be successful nurses need knowledge of and skills in the cognitive process of problem solving, commonly referred to as the Nursing Process, an understanding of the parameters of the care situation (that is the nurse and client setting), and the theoretical knowledge base needed in order to solve the problem.
>
> (Field 1987: 563)

At a theoretical level, the Nursing Process offered a 'systematic' approach to care, by drawing on assessment skills as well as nursing, biomedical and psychosocial knowledge, to plan and evaluate interventions. The basic cycle of assessment, implementation and evaluation, whilst seemingly straightforward, also offered an opportunity to deal with the expressed needs of patients, rather than dividing care into a series of tasks performed according to tradition, seniority or expertise.

Approaching nursing care in this way went against many of the traditions that had been built up since the inception of modern British nursing in the late 19th century. Whilst this book explores the impact of the Nursing Process in different cultures and settings, the British situation is marked by the lack of evaluative research on the Nursing Process, or the impact it had on nursing or health care more generally. This is surprising given that it was so widely promoted during the 1970s and early 1980s.

The Nursing Process reflected ideologies of holism in health care – values that were also being promoted at the time (Levine 1971). The growing remit of the publicly funded Health Service, however, was also undergoing repeated management restructures during the 1970s and 1980s, which meant that it was a challenging time to establish lasting change (Dingwall et al 1993). Successive British governments had weak majorities during the 1970s, which resulted in repeated cycles of change and health workers having to respond to shifting political agendas.

In the USA, Virginia Henderson claimed the Nursing Practice Acts required renewed clarity and a definition of the essence of nursing – something that the Nursing Process helped to provide. British nursing has a tradition of adopting American developments, rather than looking for inspiration from European neighbours. Together with nursing diagnoses, which arose from the emphasis placed on assessment in this new philosophy, nurse academics felt encouraged to claim that the nursing role was now distinguishable from that of medicine (Field 1987). The role that nursing claimed was focused on the helping role – assisting people to cope with the demands of illnesses that were diagnosed and treated by doctors (Henderson 1982). Such claims contributed to the professionalization project in which some were engaged (Dingwall and MacIntosh 1978). To appreciate the scale of change, it is necessary to consider the historical roots of British nursing.

HISTORICAL INFLUENCES

St Bartholomew's Hospital, in the heart of the City of London, was founded in the year 1123 as a place where the sick and infirm could find sanctuary under the care of members of a male religious order. Food and prayers were, however, usually the only interventions on offer at the time (Yeo 1995). Support for such institutions came from charitable donations or endowments from wealthy Londoners. After almost five centuries, the first physicians and surgeons were appointed at Bart's, but it was to be another 750 years before nurses were first recognized as a distinct group with specific responsibilities.

Florence Nightingale founded the first School of Nursing at nearby St Thomas' Hospital in 1860. Seven years later, St Bartholomew's Hospital established its own training school and probationer nurses were given 'instructions' for a period of 12 months. The Matron at this time was Mrs Frances Drake, the wife of a solicitor, who was not herself a trained nurse. She is said to have treated nurses rather like domestic servants; recruiting them from lower working class backgrounds and expecting them to carry heavy loads without complaint. Florence Nightingale also appeared sympathetic to the value of docility on the part of nurses: '[Nurses should] devote themselves wholly to labour on behalf of the sick and never think they were overworked or unfairly treated' (Yeo 1995: 32).

Historical accounts illustrate the importance placed on the task-based approach to nursing from earliest times. For example, Matilda Jenkins, one of the first probationer nurses at St Bartholomew's Hospital in the 1870, tells of her first days on Harley Ward:

> One day a sweep was brought into Harley with six fractured ribs. 'Pro', said Sister, 'go and wash that patient'. I had never before been shown how to set about such a task, and his hair alone, which was full of soot, nearly drove me to despair. Another day I was ordered to give soap-and-water injections to the same man, and also to a man with a fractured neck of femur. I had never given one before, and had no instructions whatever given to me. I was in tears before I had finished, and so, I fear, were the patients.
>
> (Yeo 1995: 33)

With time, nurse education passed from being the responsibility of senior medical staff (who gave lectures or demonstrations to nursing students) to experienced clinical nurses known as 'sister tutors'. By the 1930s, such appointments were common throughout the UK.

Historical accounts emphasize the many rules, regulations and traditions that had shaped nursing in UK hospitals at this time. Uniforms were elaborate, with various adornments, such as cuffs, hats or collars, used to denote rank and seniority. Nursing badges often included symbols of relevance to the institution in which nurses had trained. Nurses from The Edinburgh Royal Infirmary, for example, were known as 'Pelicans' as the fable of the pelican plucking feathers from its breast to feed its young on its own blood had been adopted as the philanthropic symbol of the hospital.

The Nurses Registration Act of 1919 set up the first national Register of Nurses. However, tradition and custom continued to shape nursing, even when senior nurses found themselves more closely involved in management roles as a result of NHS restructuring during the 1970s.

The relative youth of modern-day nursing is an important point in relation to the focus of this chapter. Nursing helped to shape, and was in turn shaped by, the traditions of the great British metropolitan hospitals, many of which were built during the Victorian era. Hospital nursing was assuming greater importance, and more complicated forms of surgery and other treatments placed greater demands on nurses' time. As hospitals became busier, so their organization moved closer to those methods used in industry, such as clear lines of authority. Coping with an increasingly complex workload further encouraged task and routine-based approaches to nursing. Reverby (1987) describes the beginnings of hospital nursing research in the USA during the 1920s and 1930s, with time and efficiency measures being applied to nursing procedures. It is also claimed that enthusiasm for such early research dwindled, as it was felt to reflect values of industry and medical science rather than nursing itself.

British nursing was also being influenced by developments overseas, primarily those taking place during the early 20th century in the USA. Whilst schools of nursing had been established in universities there since the early years of the 20th century, it was not until 1956 that the first British Department of Nursing was established at the University of Edinburgh. The bulk of nurse education in Britain continued to be located in hospital Schools of Nursing until the mid-1990s, when nurse education was finally transferred into the university sector.

Developments in the USA continued to impact on the British situation. Nurse academics, such as Virginia Henderson who taught nursing at Columbia University from 1931 until 1948, were influential in promoting the 'systematic approach' to nursing that focused attention on individual health needs, rather than nursing tasks. What may appear now as a relatively simple shift in thinking eventually resulted in a redefinition of nursing itself and how it should be delivered.

One of the most fundamental changes was that nurses were encouraged to *assess* patients' individual needs. They were then expected to *plan* care and choose between a range of alternatives about the most appropriate interventions. Thereafter, they were encouraged to *judge* the effectiveness of their actions. All of this was to be documented in written records that were updated regularly. Theoretically, any nurse with adequate expertise should be able to continue to deliver appropriate care simply by referring to the care plan available.

By assessing, planning and evaluating, nurses had adopted a rational style of decision-making most commonly seen in the diagnostic function of medicine (Crow 1995). Assessment, in particular, involved reasoning skills to highlight priorities. Encouraging nurses to work in this way resulted in the need to consider the importance of decision-making skills in this choice-based approach. As a result, a body of theory and research, never previously applied to practice-based occupations such as nursing, suddenly assumed greater relevance (albeit primarily in academic circles).

NURSES AS DECISION-MAKERS

The latter half of the 20th century saw a growing interest in research into the human capacity to assess information and make judgements from a range of competing alternatives. For instance, Eddy, in 1984, argued that cognitive processes used within applied disciplines, such as nursing or medicine, could be subjected to the same analysis as any other human activity. Decision-making research grew in importance at the same time as the Nursing Process was being promoted during the 1970s and early 1980s.

Viewing decision-making in nursing as a series of straightforward cognitive steps (involving assessment, implementation and evaluation) actually belies the complexity of the task. Whilst some clinical decisions may be relatively straightforward, others may present a series of possible alternatives. Resource or ethical implications may also compound difficulties in decision-making. One approach put forward to promote an increased understanding of decision-making is reflective practice (Schon 1991). Central to this is an appreciation of the role of intuitive reasoning:

> When we go about the spontaneous intuitive performance of the actions of everyday life, we show ourselves to be knowledgeable in a special way. Often we cannot say what it is that we know. When we try to describe it, we find ourselves at a loss or we produce descriptions that are obviously inappropriate. Our knowing is ordinarily tacit, implicit in our patterns of action and in our feel for the stuff with which we are dealing. It seems right to say that our knowing is *in* our action.
>
> (Schon 1991: 69)

Promoting insight into decision-making processes, however, also requires an appreciation of techniques that may be employed to help professionals. Newell and Simon (1972), who postulated the concept of bounded rationality, provide a useful starting point. They emphasized the limited human capacity for rational thought and the need to process decisions in turn, select relevant information with care and represent problems in simplified ways in order to reach satisfactory outcomes. Such processes may involve writing information down and selecting possible actions (both of which processes were required in assessment and care planning). This breaks decisions into manageable chunks, and results in a clinical or care hypothesis (such as a medical or nursing diagnosis). A range of methods, such as verbalizing the thinking processes involved, has been used to explore these activities.

This view of decision-making emphasizes the information-processing ability of the person involved. In practice, however, some problems are easier to solve than others. The more complex the situation, the more numerous and less accurate are likely to be the hypotheses obtained. Elstein et al (1978) explored physicians' decision-making as they talked through a series of clinical scenarios. The research suggested that a small number of core hypotheses were generated early in clinical encounters that were based on initial assessment information. These would then be accepted or rejected when matched against further clinical information. All sources of data were eventually combined with the individual clinician's ability to arrive at an accurate judgement about the patient's needs. Accuracy, therefore, depended on the relevance of the information gathered as well as the cognitive skills of the clinicians involved.

This process, termed diagnostic reasoning, was classified into the following four main stages.

- Cue acquisition and data gathering: using history taking and physical examination.
- Hypothesis generation: alternative problem patterns are retrieved from memory.
- Cue interpretation: data are interpreted in the light of the hypotheses being constructed.
- Hypothesis evaluation; data are weighted and aggregated to accept or reject the diagnostic hypothesis. If rejected, new data will be gathered to generate novel hypotheses.

The above approach emphasizes the clinician primarily as a processor of information. To an extent, this is reasonable, as there are important cognitive skills underpinning clinical decision-making. When the complexities of health care are considered, however, it is apparent that a number of additional factors impact on decision-making processes. These may include local factors, such as choices expressed by the patient, as well as more objective influences, such as resource constraints.

Each step in the diagnostic reasoning model relates to the Nursing Process cycle. Essentially, the Nursing Process, and the documentation system used in practice to record priorities, were cognitive tools to encourage nurses to think through their actions. Their everyday use, however, could not guarantee a more considered or individual approach to practice.

Indeed, during the 1980s, care planning gradually became standardized, with 'core care plans' being devised for use with patients with similar conditions or undergoing standard treatments. Far from promoting individualized care, it could be argued that the core care plan approach promoted a form of 'cookbook' nursing that detracted somewhat from the original aims of identifying and responding to individual need. Whilst evaluation could still take place by considering the effectiveness of an individual or core care plan, clinical nurses were also beginning to question the importance of additional influences, such as intuitive judgement and experience, which also seemed to impact on success in clinical situations (Benner and Wrubel 1982, Benner 1984).

THE PSYCHOLOGICAL CONTINUUM OF DECISION-MAKING

Hammond (1978) considers the full range of cognitive strategies that can be employed when problem solving occurs. This ranges from the purely rational at one extreme to the more intuitive at the other. Which one is more likely to be employed in clinical settings will depend on a variety of factors, including the complexity of the decision, the skills and expertise of those involved, and the range of options available. An example of a purely rational approach to decision-making is reflected in the use of decision trees or algorithms that map treatment choices (Dowie and Elstein 1991). Experts in the field usually derive the data to construct such models from clinical databases, published sources of evidence or subjective estimates. Statistical probabilities can be used to support this approach.

Hamm et al (1984) argues that, in normal circumstances, most problem-solving cannot be considered wholly analytical or intuitive. Instead, it is more likely to lie somewhere in between. This 'quasi-rational' approach switches between the different modes of thinking at different points in the decision-making process. An example may be a nurse consultant teaching students conducting a clinical round. Students may first be invited to offer rational or analytical cues to reach a decision about a patient's needs, and then be encouraged to temper these against more intuitive thinking about other relevant issues involved, such as levels of family support or other coexisting conditions.

The most 'analytical' mode of decision-making relates to the highly objective standard of scientific experiments, whilst intuitive judgements occur independently of peer support or technical aids. Between these lies the randomized controlled trial (currently considered the gold standard for assessing the effectiveness of new treatments in medicine), the quasi-experiment, system-aided methods and peer-aided judgements. These intermediate modes of decision-making focus on analytical methods, which are assumed to increase accuracy and reduce the influence of human error or individual bias. However, as Hamm (1984: 438) has suggested:

> Whilst the usual conditions for the acquisition of medical knowledge involve epistemological safeguards at modes 1, 2 and 3, the usual condition for its application in the clinic involve mode 6 (uncriticised private judgements), and mode 5 (group discussion) . . .

Nursing decisions are unlikely to be supported by empirical knowledge from a purely rational, experimental dimension (as much of nursing practice remains untested). The importance of qualitative evidence in nursing reflects an interest in the impact of illness, as much as the means of its resolution (Leininger 1985). Experience and intuition, therefore, also assume significance in the reality of nursing practice (Watson 1994). Intuitive judgements may be influenced by personal beliefs unique to each clinician (such as being aware of the latest empirical research or personal preferences for a specific wound dressing).

System-aided judgements are also relevant as they underpin many novel evidence dissemination methods, such as published databases being made available in the clinical setting. Care pathways also reflect a similar approach, as the choices available to clinicians are mapped out in advance, with any deviation requiring justification. The primary rationale for this approach is the control of costs, as well as ensuring consistency in standards of care across a health care economy (Tudor Hart 1998).

An additional mode of practice, which is important in the context of health care practice, is missing from Hammond's model. This involves ritualistic practice, an approach that may also be applied by practitioners from any professional group. Challenging its influence lies behind recent developments to promote awareness of clinical effectiveness and evidence-based practice, and to raise standards in the British NHS using processes of accreditation and peer-review (Coulter 1999).

Each of the above suggests that there is a 'right' way to make decisions about a patient's needs, but Fowler (1997) argues:

> Sometimes, nursing may be problem orientated or diagnosis related, but in many cases, clinicians must make health-enhancing or caring-oriented judgements about how to 'be with' the client. The term clinical reasoning most accurately describes nurse's thinking, which is situation bound and not always diagnostic in nature. Clinical reasoning involves an interaction among an individual's cognition, the subject matter, and the context of the situation where thinking occurs...from previous research it is unclear whether nurses find the Nursing Process or hypothetico-deductive models of clinical judgement useful in ambiguous reasoning tasks such as care planning.
>
> (Fowler 1997: 351)

Reasoning skills, the Nursing Process, reflective practice and evidence based care are ways to improve standards of care. Each depends on the other, however, and the lack of empirical research into the ways nurses develop care planning skills supports the need to explore these issues in future research (Fowler 1997).

THE PROFESSIONAL LEGACY OF THE NURSING PROCESS

In the UK, the main professionalizing base of nursing is located in professional organizations, such as the Royal College of Nursing, as well as the academic sector. Melia (1984, 1987) has argued that task allocation, far from being merely historical tradition, is also an appropriate means of delivering care by breaking it into chunks, and allocating these to clinicians of appropriate levels of experience and skill. An example of this may be a ward sister facing an inconsistent level of competence in the student nurses working in a given clinical area on any given day. Rather than assigning the total care of patients to these individuals, tasks may be allocated on the basis of their expected level of complexity.

The usual approach taken in British hospitals was to assign a nurse to help patients wash or undertake routine observations, another to deal with surgical dressings, whilst the most senior nurse assumed responsibility for medicines and liaising with the medical staff. This was (and still is, most probably) the reality of a functioning public health care system. Given the recent difficulties in recruiting applicants to nurse training, and concerns of the clinical competency about some of those who are qualifying, it is unlikely that the Nursing Process (in the purest sense) would be suitable for clinical areas functioning under considerable pressure, and with variable levels of competent staff (Kelly et al 2002). This is likely to be especially relevant in inner-city areas in Britain, where increased living costs add to the difficulties of educating and recruiting experienced nurses (Gould et al 2004).

Academics do not have day-to-day responsibility for care delivery in such circumstances, yet may be dismayed when clinicians do not readily adopt philosophies, models or attitudes espoused by them. Any cynicism that may have existed among practising nurses about the Nursing Process, however, was not explored systematically at the time of its implementation in Britain. This suggests that its potential and implementation may have detracted from the need to evaluate its usefulness. A possible explanation is that the Nursing Process offered a means of promoting a professionalizing ideal, as well as addressing the need to develop a more individualized approach to nursing and health care more generally. American nursing, in general, was already held in high esteem in Britain owing to the rapid expansion of graduate programmes, higher salaries and its apparently enhanced status. The Nursing Process may have been seen as an aspirational ideal for a rather disgruntled profession during the 1970s (Dingwall et al 1993).

De la Cuesta (1983) traces the most significant moment of impact for the Nursing Process in the USA to the mid-1970s when the Joint Commission on the Accreditation of Hospitals required hospitals to produce care plans in order to qualify for income from reimbursement or Federal income schemes. At this point, the Nursing Process passed from being simply a professional ideal to a political tool. Care planning allowed each item of expenditure to be accounted for and, more importantly, justified (Gubrium 1980, Gubrium and Buckholdt 1982). Care planning soon became an 'administrative art' – some way removed from the idealized original goal of improving the quality of care by systematically enhancing the diagnostic reasoning approach to nursing.

In Britain, the Nursing Process was first discussed in the nursing press during the mid-1970s. By 1977, it was being promoted in the general hospital sector (de la Cuesta 1983). Once again, its initial champions were academics and nurse teachers who saw its potential for promoting idealized approaches to nursing. In 1977, it was incorporated into the syllabus for general nurse training and, in 1979, a British author published the first book on the subject. The rapidity of implementation suggests that the Nursing Process was highly significant to nurses and policy makers of the time. It is unusual for a nursing philosophy to be adopted so rapidly and on such a grand scale. The nursing elite clearly must have believed it offered more than a systemic approach for delivering nursing care.

Given this state of affairs, it is surprising that the Nursing Process was not subjected to closer scrutiny. One study conducted by Hayward at King's College, London, in 1986 reviewed available evidence and sought the views of key stakeholders. Few examples of successful implementation could be identified and the conclusion was drawn that further consultation should have taken place before such a significant change had been set in motion. De la Cuesta (1983) further examined the implementation of the Nursing Process in British and American hospitals using interviews and observations of practice. She suggested that nursing histories were being sought but were then used mainly as reference points, rather than the source for reaching a plan of care. Care plans would commonly emphasize medical procedures and physical tasks dominated. Interestingly, despite the effort involved in their production, nursing care plans were not always valued by hospitals, and were routinely destroyed at the time of discharge or death (unlike medical notes that were considered legal documents). The emphasis placed on physical care reflects its dominance in many settings, whereas psycho-social support may not have been so easy to commit to paper. The language of the Nursing Process was also heavily derivative from medicine (using terms such as 'prescriptions' of nursing care and 'nursing diagnoses'). Such terms never really caught on in Britain and appeared to achieve little in terms of the status of most practising nurses. Dingwall et al (1993: 217) term this language a form of 'ideological hegemony', which threatened to produce 'a common occupational culture dominated by general nursing'.

Whilst the language of the Nursing Process may have been more readily adopted into the health care culture of the USA, few British nurses appeared to employ it outside academic circles. Its impact on contemporary nursing in this country appears to have been minimal.

TOWARDS SOME CONCLUSIONS

In light of the above, it is difficult to judge the overall benefits of the Nursing Process fairly. In Britain it did focus attention on new areas of research, such as decision-making and clinical expertise. This, in turn, probably contributed to the recognition of nursing as an important player in the modernization targets set for the NHS in the late 1990s. Responsibilities that had previously been the remit of medical staff only were passed to nurses out of political expediency, as much as any attempt to meet the professionalizers' aspirations. The emergence of advanced nursing roles, such as nurse consultants, attempted to address the need for a career structure that would retain skilled nurses in the NHS (and in close proximity to patient care). Whilst undoubtedly also a political development, the nurse consultant role does seem closer to the professional ideal espoused by earlier generations of nurses. What these individuals do not appear to do, however, is to base their interventions on as formal a method as the Nursing Process. Their capacity for skilled judgement and expertise is assumed, rather than having to be detailed in written plans. Care planning itself is changing with new electronic systems promoting less laborious methods of health care documentation. Indeed, some new British hospitals are adopting electronic, interprofessional information systems with the eventual aim of becoming 'paperless'.

Perhaps the most significant legacy of the Nursing Process is its contribution to nurse education. By allowing learners to consider the needs of those in their care, it promoted a means of recognizing priorities and highlighting the importance of professional judgement. It took time, however, for attention to be paid to the equally important skills of intuition and experience. More recent developments include the application of an evidence-based approach to support care-planning decisions (Mason and Attree 1997). Questions also remain, however, about the extent to which the Nursing Process approach shielded students from the demands and realities of practice where care planning may become a time-consuming luxury (or one to be carried out in tandem with competing tasks).

The Nursing Process was undoubtedly a product of its time. De la Cuesta (1983) is one of the few to consider the coverage given to it in the nursing press at the time of its implementation. The main professional concerns included a rejection of task-based nursing, disquiet at the lack of individualized models of care, low levels of job satisfaction amongst nurses and criticism of the superficial nature of the nurse–patient relationship. It is beyond the scope of this chapter to consider the latter point in the depth it probably merits. It is important, however, to emphasize that, following the era of the Nursing Process, the concept of caring itself became a significant concern in theoretical circles (Kelly 1998). Whether the Nursing Process helped or hindered a deeper understanding of caring processes in nursing practice does not appear to have been subjected to empirical scrutiny. Seminal research by Menzies in 1963, however, did suggest that task allocation may have helped to distance nurses from suffering (and so reduce their own anxiety about the work they were involved in).

Neither is there any clear evidence, however, that care planning promoted better interpersonal communication between nurses and patients. Some models of nursing, such as the one proposed by Peplau (1990), were more encouraging of the nurse encountering the patient with a 'blank sheet of paper' philosophy rather than attempting to fit needs into predetermined categories of a particular model of nursing. Such humanistic philosophies most commonly derive from the field of mental health nursing, where physical care did not always assume such dominance.

In retrospect, the Nursing Process appears to have had most impact at the theoretical level. Clinicians took from it what was most useful (such as a method for assessing need and prioritizing care). An example of this is the way it has recently been applied to particular clinical issues, such as identifying patients at increased risk of falling (Uden et al 1999). It also provided a useful tool for students who were encouraged to consider patient care in a more holistic fashion. The attention paid to nursing models, theories and diagnoses, which were appearing at the same time, seemed to impact less in practice settings in Britain (Kennedy 1993), although they did, once again, promote further theoretical debate and research (Tierney 1998).

Philosophies of decision-making, holism and person-centredness contributed to a change in thinking about health care and how it could be delivered in a more individualized fashion. The move from task-based models of care to one in which nursing interventions were directed by assessed needs was a radical step in the development of the nursing role. As a result, novel concerns began to emerge for nursing, such as a need to appreciate the psychology of decision-making and clinical judgement. The systematic approach to nursing care was intended to foster more 'rational' or 'scientific' decision-making. Ironically, it was the more qualitative, emotional dimension of nursing work that began to be questioned – a shift which problematized the role of nursing once more.

The essence and philosophy of nursing continued to change as new and expanded roles evolved. In some areas, this resulted in the development of a counterculture to the dominant medical model. This movement has culminated in the emergence of the 'expert patients', who wish to be involved directly in planning their own care and in the decisions made about their health (Coulter 2002). This places new demands on nurses who, alongside other professional groups, must seek ways of working with patients on a more equal footing than early versions of the Nursing Process allowed. As Coulter argues:

> When patients are given the opportunity to make informed choices they usually welcome it. Unreasonable or irrational demands are not as common as many clinicians fear. Shared decision making could be one of the best ways to ensure more appropriate use of health care resources, yet professional training programmes have been slow to incorporate it or to inculcate the necessary skills. The effort and resources required are relatively modest, but the rewards for patients, clinicians and the health system as a whole could be considerable.
>
> (Coulter 2002: 47)

Facing up to such a challenge indicates how far the role of nursing in health care has changed, as well as indicating the types of changes that lie ahead. From its earliest historical roots, where a subservient role to medicine was assumed, nursing has grown in stature until it is now perceived as a central component in the delivery of effective health care. This has required the emergence of new roles and responsibilities, as well as closer involvement in clinical governance systems and research activity that has relevance to the needs of patients (Boden and Kelly 1999). Some changes can be traced to ideological shifts in thinking, such as the Nursing Process, that helped to clarify the essential role of nursing. These developments also played a part in developing a clearer sense of professional identity for nurses and nursing.

This chapter has provided an overview of the historical roots of nursing in Britain. From the establishment of the modern nursing role, those involved have promoted professional ideals, examined the theoretical basis of their skills and developed new ways of conceptualizing the nursing contribution to health care. The impact of the Nursing Process is evident in its ideological, as much as its practical, legacies. In retrospect, the Nursing Process seems to have symbolized the ambitions of nursing at a time when wider social factors were forcing it to examine its status. Understanding the impact of the Nursing Process, therefore, requires an appreciation of the social contexts in which it was developed and applied. The lessons drawn from the British context suggest that ideologies of holism and professional judgement that underpinned the Nursing Process proved more enduring in the longer term than its impact on nursing practice.

REFERENCES

Benner P 1984 From novice to expert. Addison Wesley, Menlo Park, CA

Benner P, Wrubel J 1982 Skilled clinical knowledge: the value of perceptual awareness. Nurse Education 7: 11–17

Boden L, Kelly D 1999 Clinical governance; the route to (modern, dependable) nursing research? NT Research 4: 177–188

Coulter A 1999 NICE and CHI: reducing variations and raising standards. Health Care 1999/2000. King's Fund, London

Coulter A 2002 The autonomous patient. Ending paternalism in medical care. The Nuffield Trust, London

Crow R 1995 The cognitive component of nursing assessment: an analysis. Journal of Advanced Nursing 22: 206–212

De la Cuesta C 1983 The nursing process: from development to implementation. Journal of Advanced Nursing 8: 365–371

Dingwall R, MacIntosh J (eds) 1978 Readings in the sociology of nursing. Churchill Livingstone, Edinburgh

Dingwall R, Rafferty A M, Webster C 1993 An introduction to the social history of nursing. Routledge, London

Dowie J, Elstein A 1991 Professional judgement: a reader in clinical decision making. Cambridge University Press, Cambridge

Eddy DM 1984 Variations in physician practice: the role of uncertainty. Health Affairs 3: 74–89

Elstein A, Shulman L, Sprafka S 1978 Medical problem solving: an analysis of clinical reasoning. Harvard University Press, Cambridge, MA

Field P A 1987 The impact of nursing theory on the clinical decision making process. Journal of Advanced Nursing 12: 563–571

Fowler L 1997 Clinical reasoning strategies used during care planning. Clinical Nursing Research 6: 349–361

Gould D, Carr G, Kelly D, Brown P 2004 Seconding health care assistants to a pre-registration nursing course: evaluation of a novel scheme. NT Research 9: 50–63

Gubrium J 1980 Doing care plans in patient conferences. Social Science and Medicine 14A: 659–667

Gubrium J, Buckholdt D 1982 Describing care: image and practice in rehabilitation. Oelgeschlager, Gunn & Hain, Cambridge, MA

Hamm R, Clark J, Bursztajn H 1984 Psychiatrist's theory judgements: describing and improving decision making process. Medical Decision Making 4: 425–447

Hammond K 1978 Towards increasing competence of thought in public policy formation. In: Hammond KR (ed.) Judgement and decision in public policy formation. Westview Press, Colorado

Hayward J 1986 Report of the Nursing Process Evaluation Working Group. Kings College, University of London, Nursing Education Research Unit, London

Henderson V 1982 The Nursing Process – is the title right? Journal of Advanced Nursing 7: 103–116

Kelly D 1998 Caring and cancer nursing; framing the reality using selected social science theory. Journal of Advanced Nursing 28: 728–736

Kelly D, Simpson S, Brown P 2002 An action research project to establish and evaluate the Clinical Practice Facilitator role for junior nurses in an acute hospital setting. Journal of Clinical Nursing 11: 90–98

Kennedy T 1993 Nursing models fail in practice. British Journal of Nursing 2: 133–136

Leininger M 1985 Nature, rationale, and importance of qualitative research methods in nursing. In: Leininger M (ed.) Qualitative research methods in nursing. Grune & Stratton, New York

Levine M 1971 Holistic nursing. Nursing Clinics of North America 6: 253–264

Mason G, Attree M 1997 The relationship between research and the Nursing Process in clinical practice. Journal of Advanced Nursing 26: 1045–1049

Melia K 1984 Student nurses' construction of occupational socialisation. Sociology of Health and Illness 6: 132–151

Melia K 1987 Learning and working: The occupational socialization of nurses. Tavistock, London

Menzies I 1963 A case study in the functioning of social systems as a defence against anxiety. A report of a study of the nursing service of a general hospital. Human Relations 13: 95–121

Newell A, Simon H 1972 Human problem solving. Prentice Hall, Engelwood Cliffs, NJ

Peplau H 1990 Interpersonal relations model: theoretical constructs, principles and general applications. In: Reynolds W, Cormack D (eds) Psychiatric and mental health nursing: theory and practice. Chapman and Hall, London

Reverby S 1987 A legitimate relationship: nursing, hospitals and science in the twentieth century. In: Long DE, Golden J (eds) The American general hospital. Cornell University Press, Ithaca, NY

Schon D 1991 From technical rationality to reflection in action. In: Dowie J, Elstein A (eds) Professional judgement. A reader in clinical decision making. Cambridge: Cambridge University Press

Tierney A 1998 Nursing models: extant or extinct? Journal of Advanced Nursing 18: 77–85

Tudor Hart J 1998 Expectations of health care: promoted, managed or shared? Health Expectations 1: 1–2

Uden G, Ehnfors M, Sjostrum K 1999 Use of initial risk assessment and recording as the main nursing interventions in identifying risk of falls. Journal of Advanced Nursing 29: 145–152

Watson S 1994 An exploratory study into a methodology for the examination of decision making by nurses in the clinical area. Journal of Advanced Nursing 20: 351–360

Yeo G 1995 Nursing at Bart's. A history of the nursing service and nurse education at St Bartholomew's Hospital, London. Oxford: Alden Press

Chapter **3**

The Nursing Process: nursing discourse and managerial technologies

Niels Buus and Michael Traynor

INTRODUCTION

In this chapter, we take a step back from operational issues connected with the Nursing Process. Instead of looking at its usefulness or implementation, we ask whether the Nursing Process exists at all, apart from as a kind of linguistic label that can point to almost any concept. We then explore links between the way that the Nursing Process has been discussed and a generalized drive for visibility. We argue this drive is characteristic not only of a newly invigorated managerialism, which has gained ascendancy in many countries over the last 25 years, but of a deeper cultural and philosophical urge towards ever higher degrees of visibility and order. We rehearse the argument that this desire has been apparent in Western culture since the end of the 18th century. Our approach will be to carry out an in-depth analysis of a small number of textual extracts, which exemplify particular and influential kinds of discussion about the Nursing Process. Our analytical orientation is informed by discourse analysis, particularly in its poststructuralist forms. Discourse analysis can show that what appears to be natural is usually the result of social, often linguistic, processes that work to support particular interests. Because discourse analysis promises to challenge apparently stable versions of order and identity, the approach has the potential to give rise to the idea of alternative understandings and arrangements. Once imagined, these can offer a sense of liberation to groups for whom the existing 'natural' order is experienced as oppressive. We will argue that the promotion of the Nursing Process as a natural advance in nursing practice can, inadvertently, have oppressive effects on practising nurses.

CONTEXTUAL ISSUES: NURSING PROFESSIONALISM AND THE RISE OF MANAGERIAL RATIONALITY

In many Western economies, the 1980s saw the beginning of an era of new managerialism in public services such as health and welfare. This era of stringency was at least partly a result of the downturn in the world economy in the wake of the increase in price of crude oil between 1974 and 1976. Partly it was the result of New-right governments in the UK and USA wishing to reduce the power of bodies such as trade unions and the traditional professions.

The attraction of managerialism ran deeper than such contingent responses. It touched a Western desire for intense visibility and control that has caused concern to some analysts (Adorno and Horkheimer 1979, Foucault 1980). In the early decades of the 20th century, systematic management was proposed in the USA by F. W. Taylor as the true remedy for national 'inefficiency'. It was 150 years before, that Bentham (1748–1832) had proposed the idea of the Panopticon, his annular prison design which combined total visibility – or its ever-present possibility – with efficiency and humanity (Foucault 1977). One pair of eyes could supervise the behaviour of many inmates without the need for violent punishment. The principle could be applied not only in prisons but in workhouses, schools or hospitals. The objects of such surveillance learned to discipline their own behaviour. In Western scientifically advanced countries, formal, rational and controllable industrial process and systems marked a powerful combination of technical advance and quasi-religious vision. Science provided not only a method, meticulous recording of empirical observation, but a vision of progress out of the darkness of ignorance and unreflective habit. So pervasive was this vision that no group seeking credibility could afford to ignore it.

NURSING AND THE VISION OF PROGRESS

In 19th century thought, where modern nursing originated, a number of ideas coalesced and gained an influence well beyond the end of that era, and certainly influenced the development of nursing.

The *first* was enlightenment thinking. This emerged in Europe in the previous century, articulated by the philosophical writing of, particularly, Immanuel Kant (1724–1804). He proposed that humanity faced the challenge of a coming of age, of a growing away from a childlike subjugation to the authority of religion and monarchs to a mature self-reliance. This was made possible by the use of reason, and reason was available, in egalitarian fashion, to every human being (Foucault 1984).

The *second* was evolutionary theory, or rather, evolutionary social theory. Such theorizing went far beyond Darwin's studies and focused on the notion of human and cultural progress. Aspects of and evidence for human progress were everywhere: for example, many 19th century anthropologists produced accounts of the early history of humanity in which humanity's evolution from primitive states includes the observation that 'abstract' thinking replaces 'concrete' thinking (University of Waterloo Ontario 2002).

The *third* was technological advance. Since the time of astronomical discoveries, which were made possible by technical inventions in optics, technology had enabled an ever-greater range of scientific activity and had also created national wealth, which supported this enterprise. In Britain, this advance was embodied in the industrial revolution, which, in spite of its economic benefits, many saw as leading to serious social and cultural problems. The reform of nursing arose partly as a proposed solution to increases in ill-health and poverty among the new industrial working classes.

SCIENCE/PROGRESS IN THE DISCOURSES OF NURSING

Modern nursing in the USA and Britain emerged in the midst of these influences. Nutting and Dock (1907), early historians of nursing, linked the caring that they saw nursing embodying to human evolutionary progress. Later, in the mid-20th century, the language of progress is still very much apparent in reflections on the professional status of nursing and on new technologies, such as nursing theory and the Nursing Process. Professional status was identified with progress and, as Nightingale had argued, with independence from medicine. As its drive towards professionalization became more efficient, its leaders articulated its progressive and scientific basis more strongly. Crucially, to be seen as professional, the daily practice of nursing also needed to become articulated, formalized and hence visible. What is tacit needs to become explicit if it is to have a place in the modern rational world. Johnson, probably the first nurse theorist, wrote in 1959: 'No profession can

long exist without making explicit its theoretical basis for practice . . .'
(Johnson 1959; cited in Mc Kenna 1997: 35).

In the 1980s, a number of US nursing academics published reflections on
the theoretical advances in the profession during the previous decades.
Many of these writers saw autonomous professional practice as possible
only if it could be based upon elaborate scientific theory. They describe this
as a coming of age of the profession. This move parallels Kant's telling of
the history of humanity in his essay 'Was ist Aufklärung?' [What is enlightenment?]. He both celebrates a newly acclaimed human reason, as mentioned above and recognizes its promise of emancipation from traditional
authority (Foucault 1984). In fact, the development of nursing theories is
placed explicitly within the context of Kant's account of human understanding by one nursing writer (Fawcett 1984).

The narratives woven by Fawcett (1984) and Meleis (1985) about the
efforts of nurse theorists over the past decades appear strongly influenced
by social evolutionary theory and a certain triumphalism. They described
the 1960s and 1970s as a period characterized by the development of nursing
theories and models. The impetus for such an enterprise was the desire to
forge a range of 'concepts' that were distinct from those employed within
medicine and to disentangle them from those of other disciplines. As previously mentioned, 'abstract thinking' was seen as an advance from the
realm of the practical. This change in nursing is presented in their writing
as a heroic 'journey' with 'stages' and 'milestones' (Meleis 1985: 7), as a
development, an advance, an 'evolution of nursing', its champions heralded
as 'pioneering' (Fawcett 1984: viii). The establishment in 1955 of the journal
Nursing Research is described as the first significant 'milestone' in nursing
after Florence Nightingale, offering 'confirmation that nursing is indeed a
scientific discipline and that its progress will depend on whether or not
nurses pursue truth through an avenue that respectable disciplines pursue,
namely research' (Meleis 1985: 13). Indeed, the era of theory building is seen
as the culmination of the history of nursing. It is seen as the epitome of a
kind of thinking that Kant's humanity come of age must achieve.

PROCESS/PROGRESS IN THE DISCOURSES OF NURSING

From this perspective, the Nursing Process has the simple advantage of
allowing the potentially endless and uncontrollable variety of activities,
which constitute day-to-day nursing to be formalized, made visible by their
manner of recording, and hence legitimized within a broad scientific discourse. We now go on to analyse the early development of the Nursing
Process.

A SKETCH FOR A DISCOURSE ANALYSIS OF THE NURSING PROCESS

A discourse of nursing

Foucault advocated strongly for an analysis of discourse that avoided a
hermeneutic exegesis of what is said. Foucault wanted to open a field of
inquiry where the naked statement is the starting point for analysis. Rather

than exploring a deeper meaning of what is said, he searched for regularities among directly observable statements. These regularities are named discourses or discursive formations that construe areas of knowledge, in particular, rule-bound patterns. It might be confusing that 'discourse' can both denote a particular field of knowledge and the regularities making these fields of knowledge possible. Discourses are not authored by speaking subjects but are autonomous entities governing what one can say and think at any time in history: 'One cannot speak of anything at any time' (Foucault 1972: 44). In this sense, our ideas and our knowledge, which seem novel and creative for us, are generated continuously by discursive regularities. This means that what we express through language is both made possible and constricted by discourse. Thus, the analysis of discourse is an attempt to outline the discursive regularities in order to outline the limits of our knowledge: to point at its limits and the historical and institutional contingencies of what we know. In this part of the chapter, we will outline a discourse of nursing and point at how the Nursing Process becomes part of these regularities.

It would be premature and perhaps misleading to talk about 'the discourse of the Nursing Process', as the phrase indicates an individualizable discursive coherency round 'the Nursing Process'. A more fertile approach, in discourse analytic terms, is to start by regarding the Nursing Process as a discursive object, which is being picked up and transformed by discourses that are situated in non-discursive contexts. A discursive object is something taken up by language and given a verbal form. In this section we will examine the ways the Nursing Process is situated in nursing discourses.

The 'two processes'

According to Henderson (1987), the term 'Nursing Process' was coined in the late 1950s. It appeared in the work of nursing scholars at the Yale School of Nursing, who were interested in the psychosocial aspects of health care. These nurses and their collaborators recognized a therapeutic potential of communication and interpersonal relations. They described the collaborative striving of the patient and the nurse towards healing in terms of a process. In the mid-1970s, however, this conceptualization of a process was challenged by a group of nursing scholars at the Catholic University of America. These scholars described a process more in line with a biomedical and science-based research process: identifying problems, planning, implementation and evaluation (Henderson 1987). The difference between these two conceptualizations of the Nursing Process seems at first glance substantial, as it inverts the strategies of professional recognition and status, including not least the interdisciplinary boundary with biomedicine. The Yale nurses regarded the psychosocial process as a central part of a valid platform on which to differentiate nursing from biomedicine. After the reconceptualization, such a disciplinary and professional platform is developed by copying successful biomedical techniques, such as diagnosis and plans for treatment; cf. the analysis of nursing diagnoses by Powers (2002). In this perspective, the two conceptualizations appear as opposites.

The conceptualization of a – or *the* – Nursing Process has, since the birth of the term, been discussed and elaborated by nursing scholars; this interest and debate is reflected in an enormous body of literature on the topic. In 1996, Varcoe analysed a number of critiques of the Nursing Process. She concludes that there is no conceptual consensus about *what the Nursing Process is* and *what it is for* (Varcoe 1996). However, indirectly her analysis offers a rather disheartening interpretation of the notion of the Nursing Process: it would seem that the Nursing Process has become immune to serious critique through the inclusion of a range of theoretical variations and added *ad hoc* hypotheses.

In order to avoid the seemingly impossible project of coming to terms with what the Nursing Process is, we adopt a discourse analytic approach towards it. We regard the notion of 'the Nursing Process', as an empty or a floating signifier: The meaning of the Nursing Process is contingent on the articulatory practices surrounding a discourse (cf. Laclau and Mouffe 1985, Foucault 1991). This means, for instance, that the differences between the way the Nursing Processes is referred to by Henderson, Varcoe and others must be conceptualized as part of different discourses, such as the humanities and social sciences vs. medical sciences. Our aim is firstly to contextualize the articulations and meanings of the Nursing Processes within nursing discourses and secondly to contextualize the process within wider societal notions of managerialism. We will argue that the differences between the 'Yale Nursing Process' and the 'Catholic University Nursing Process' both reflect continuities and discontinuities in the way nurses talk about practice. The latter appear in the ways that the process is interpreted and used by societal forces outside nursing (Latimer 1995, Purkis 1999).

Above we outlined Henderson's account of a major change in how the Nursing Process was conceptualized. We argued that the reformulation of the Nursing Process repositioned it within nursing discourses so that it became part of a strategy for professional recognition, but it would be hasty to assume it was also a significant discursive change within nursing.

In her seminal work on the discourse of the nursing profession in 20th-century Denmark, Beedholm detects a set of discursive regularities in the production, adoption and integration of theory into the nursing texts (Beedholm 2003). She does this by analysing Denmark's single professional nursing journal as well as the general Danish nursing textbooks published throughout the century. The attempt is to identify thresholds between fundamental discursive changes and more superficial fluctuations. Crudely summing up the findings, and ignoring the subtle differences between various positions in the field of nursing, the most pervasive and central discursive rules are as follows.

- *Normativization: the descriptive becomes normative.* What is accepted as normative changes and expands through time. Early in the last century, the normative was a demand on the nurse's external behaviour and the right manner of nursing. Later it becomes less articulated but comprises a conscious reflection on thoughts and values. The scope of normativism now includes the nurse's interior; the nurse's self and professional identity.

- *Instrumentalization: increased understanding becomes an instrument for intervention*. Instrumentalization also changes through time. Early in the century the nursing situation is described as *the* intervention. Later the nurses' thoughts and feelings are conceptualized as instrumental means to improve the outcome of their nursing actions.
- *Sliding: differences between levels of abstraction and between types of theory are ignored*. Differences between scientific practice and everyday life are ignored. Practice adopts characteristics of research at the same time as research is equalized to everyday practice.

All in all, these regular processes create fairly homogeneous theories (Beedholm 2003). Beedholm's study is concerned with a limited set of textual genres: the professional writings. A discourse analysis of other nursing documents may point to different rules of formation, as the journal and the books are authored by nurses with particular education or positions, namely the nursing scholars. In light of the discursive rules identified by Beedholm, the difference between the two conceptualizations of the Nursing Process, respectively from Yale University and The Catholic University, becomes less significant. This point can be illustrated by two extracts from Henderson's paper. Firstly, Henderson cites from the Yale nurse Orlando's *The dynamic nurse patient relationship*:

> The purpose of nursing is to supply the help a patient requires in order for his needs to be met. The nurse achieves her purpose by initiating a process which ascertains the patient's immediate need and helps to meet the need directly or indirectly.
>
> (Orlando in Henderson 1987: 15)

In this quote all three rules seem to be operating: the normative impetus for action, the drive from understanding to intervention, and an indirect sliding between the science of psychodynamics and everyday nursing practice.

Secondly, turning towards the Catholic University conception of the Nursing Process:

> nursing is said to be 'the process . . . of determining the client's problems, making plans to solve them, initiating the plan or assigning others to implement it, and evaluating the extent to which the plan was effective in resolving the problem identified'.
>
> (Henderson 1987: 13)

Here, the normative impetus is analogous to the one above: there is a problem (need) to be solved (met). The process, knowledge of the process, is an organizing instrument for the nurse. Further, there is a distinct resemblance between a rational research process and this formulation of the systematic problem-oriented Nursing Process. This outer resemblance creates a double slide between types of theory. On the one hand, it allows the verbalization of scientific concepts etc. as concepts *about* practice, and on the other hand practice is *brought close to* science; pulling science and practice towards each other, diminishing their differences. This juxtaposition of the processes, based on Henderson's illustrative quotes, shows that both conceptualizations of the Nursing Process are closely linked to the discursive regularities of nursing identified by Beedholm. This link suggests that both processes are part of the same system of thought despite their superficial differences. There are also discontinuities. These seem to be associated with the particular way nursing discourse is articulated and how these articulations resemble discourses from outside nursing.

PROCESSING DISCURSIVE ELEMENTS THROUGH THE NURSING PROCESS

It is not sufficient to regard the Nursing Process as simply a discursive object; it is also an active process *giving rise to* discursive objects. Even though both the Yale University and the Catholic University Nursing Processes resonate perfectly with the central regularities of nursing discourse, they differ in the ways in which they relate to other discursive elements.

Both versions of the processes establish a logical link between someone with a deficit that (directly or indirectly) is relieved by a nurse. These objects are articulated differently according to the specific discourse. (We, of course, do not hold a privileged position outside discourse and 'someone', 'deficit' and 'nurse' reflect our choices in naming of the objects.) Looking at the two extracts from Henderson's paper one can observe Orlando talking about a 'patient', 'his needs' and a female 'nurse'. The patient's needs are ascertained by the nurse and then relieved through the process. In this sense, the identification of a need and the means to meet it are mediated by the nurse–patient process. By way of contrast, The Catholic University nurses talk of a 'client', 'problems' and only implicitly about someone doing nursing. The agent is written out of the sentence; the agent of nursing, someone doing nursing, has been removed, indicating a different way of articulating nursing compared to Orlando's view. This way of using a passive sentence structure is a characteristic of medical discourse, see for instance, Lane and Lawler (2003) for a short and powerful introduction and critique of medical discourse. Here problems are determined (by someone doing nursing), plans are made to solve them, plans are implemented and the effectiveness of the plan is evaluated. In this articulation of a Nursing Process, problems are logically linked with plans to solve them; and the plans are implemented and their effectiveness evaluated. Thus, the agent carrying out the nursing actions is hardly present in this conception of a Nursing Process: the agent is either 'written out' or the acts are conceptualized as plans rather than actions suggesting, maybe, that the conception is concerned with matters beyond the individual nurse.

In a very basic way, the links between the set of discursive objects: the patient, a deficit and a (present) nurse, justifies the nurse's professional mandate; cf. Dingwall and Allen (2001). Therefore, it is probably possible to find a 'Nursing Process' in any nursing theory: Duldt offers a list of variations of the Nursing Process inherent in different nursing theories, including, apparently, that even Florence Nightingale used the process – obviously unknowingly (Duldt 1995).

In the name of a Nursing Process, the basic configuration of discursive objects can be theorized in a variety of ways, which are not mutually exclusive, probably because they basically are part of the same discourse. The two processes, one from Yale University and one from the Catholic University, therefore, can be stuck together in the same model by just adding Yale conceptions of interpersonal relations, even notions of holism, to the process of identifying problems in the Catholic University model. This was how one of this chapter's authors first encountered the process in the early 1990s, necessitating doublethink in an Orwellian sense: *Doublethink* means the power of holding two contradictory beliefs in one's mind simultaneously, and accepting both of them.

Not only can the two models be combined, a range of objects, processes or technologies can be added to the basic structure, such as nursing diagnoses (Powers 2002) or reflective practice (Heath 1998). These two objects differ, however, in the sense that they have different affinities to the two processes: In this sense, there *are* two 'discourses of the Nursing Process', two discursive regularities around two different Nursing Processes. Heath argues that reflective practice should be conceptualized as part of the Nursing Process partly because it is concerned with nursing practice 'as it is'. Such an argument can be read as an attempt to rehabilitate the individual nurse's ability to think, which in at least the Catholic University model seems not to be an issue. Again, the approach is in line with the above identified nursing discourse, and can be seen as an attempt to 'doublethink' the two models. We suggest that a lot of the polemics surrounding the Nursing Process is related to 'doublethinking' at least two different conceptions of the Nursing Process simultaneously. The conceptualization of nursing diagnoses differs from that of reflective practice. Nursing diagnoses are a technology that fits the distancing logic of the Catholic University Nursing Process like a hand in a glove: it merely extends its basic configuration of discursive objects by giving a name to the client's problem. This process of naming and casting light on problems, and having a standardized approach to solving them belongs to a discourse pervading society far beyond nursing, given just one expression in managerialism (Traynor 1999).

To sum up, even though the two conceptions of a process can be interpreted as being part of the same discourse of nursing, they differ in the way they articulate and organize a basic structure of discursive objects. We have tried to outline tentatively these discursive continuities and discontinuities. The shift of conceptualization is significant, in spite of both being part of mainstream nursing discourse, as the Catholic University Nursing Process has a higher affinity towards managerial discourses and technologies. The specific adoption of the Nursing Process within managerial discourses is discussed below.

VISIBILITY AND METHODS FOR RECORDING WORK

We now discuss two published papers that explore the double-edged promise of various recording systems to render the work of nurses visible. The promise is double-edged because, as both papers argue, this visibility brings an unwitting transformation of their work. Papers by Purkis (1999) and Latimer (1995) are unusual among the large number of texts discussing the Nursing Process, in that they decentre nursing work, and place it into the context of rising managerialism and accountability in health care systems around the world. Their papers are also exceptional in their refusal to make normative statements (cf. Beedholm 2003, cited above) about nursing practice. Linked to this, both are antiessentialist, in that they do not start from an assumption that nursing work has an essential nature that needs expression, protection or rediscovery. Both draw on actor network theory and the work of Latour to explore how humans and non-human technologies work together to achieve certain social and political accomplishments (Latour 1987, 1991).

Purkis (1999) argues that particular historical contingencies combine to create a situation where the interests of managerialism and professionalism become aligned, in surprising ways that are not immediately apparent. In Purkis' case study, a group of nurses are setting up an innovative community-based service. For political reasons, their professional body, the Registered Nurses Association of British Columbia (RNABC), emphasizes the need for the service not only to establish its novel nature but to reassure an anxious medical association that the full scope of nursing practice in this situation does not stray over what it sees as the boundary into medical work. Therefore, the way that this particular practice would be recorded, and hence, represented, was crucial, and clearly not a neutral technological detail. The RNABC had an interest in showing what the 'full scope of practice' could look like when it was freed from the constraints of institutionalized hospital health care delivery. (The present authors understand 'full scope of practice' to suggest a state when nursing is able to achieve its true nature and potential – its *telos*.) Purkis writes as one of the members of a team hired to evaluate this new service. She acknowledges that she too was 'enrolled', or drawn in on the ground of having an interest in producing 'an account of nursing practice that was innovative and new' (Purkis 1999: 150). She advised the team to adopt a recording system that would not, in her own uneasy term 'disguise' the true nature of the work undertaken. As it happened, her advice was not heeded and the nursing minimum dataset (NMDS) was the recording system adopted for the project.

In times of financial stringency, all health care practitioners become conscious of their vulnerability (Pollitt 1993, Hunter 1994). Those advocating the dissemination of the NMDS call on these powerful anxieties: 'We need nursing information to help articulate our contribution to the health of Canadians' (Anderson et al 1994, in Purkis 1999: 151).

One response is to learn how to 'speak the manager's language', as many in nursing have urged their colleagues (Prentice 1991, Traynor 1999). The apparent benefits are many:

- nurses grow in confidence as they learn to 'articulate' what they do;
- they grow in solidarity as the language of this articulation is standardized;
- they become conscious of the notion of cost effectiveness in the face of skill-mix and downsizing;
- they become inhabitants of the modern, rational world.

Purkis notes that the articulation of an argument to adopt managerialist language marks the moment of the alignment of managerial and professional interests. She argues that in this moment of alignment, which enacts a desire for visibility in managerialist terms, nursing work is transformed from what she calls 'naked desire to care for the sick and injured' (Purkis 1999: 151) into managerialist statements based on the value of context-free information. It is because the technologies of managerialism are not neutral that nurses and patients alike are transformed, not merely innocently recorded. To repeat the crucial point Purkis makes, nurses actively participate in this transformation (rather than being compelled to do so) in a desire to emphasize their professional identity and specifically to align themselves to a newly emerged managerialism. In the event, the nurses in her case study attempted to run two parallel recording systems. One, the Omaha system, required them to tick any relevant category such as 'presenting problem'. These were then to be entered into a computer database. The second was a more open-ended narrative. The nurses reported, however, that the Omaha system was not helping them to approach practice systematically or holistically. They were frustrated by a lack of categories to record their interactions adequately and also became uneasy about 'discrepancies' between what the two systems recorded. The approach became burdensome and some nurses turned away from reading the notes entirely, saying it was more useful simply to ask the patients why they had come.

In the second paper, Latimer starts from a similar position to Purkis, arguing that the Nursing Process is not a neutral technology. Rather it is 'based on a particular model of human action: an information-processing, problem-solving model which assumes the possibility that cognitions can be detached from other issues' (Latimer 1995: 214).

More than this, Latimer argues that it is common for analysts to claim that nurses have 'failed' to live up to the normative intentions of the Nursing Process through various forms of incomplete implementation. The notion of 'incomplete implementation' derives from a particular model used to attempt to understand the uptake of innovations. Rogers (1985) proposed a diffusion model of the uptake of innovation. This is an approach that has become a 'common-sense' explanation in which knowledge of the benefits of an innovation spread among potential implementers. Full and early uptake is the ideal from which any 'deviations' need to be explained. Latimer argues that the Nursing Process, like other innovations (e.g. primary nursing, patient participation) has been 'loaded with positive value'. Nurses' behaviour becomes one of a range of variables that explain the supposed poor uptake of the Nursing Process (or processes). This common conception that the Nursing Process has rarely, if ever, been completely achieved hampers any attempt to evaluate its impact on the care that nurses deliver to patients, and hence, on patient outcomes. Nevertheless, such recording systems as contained in the Nursing Process begin to define what is 'normal' practice in such a way that deviations from the norm can be identified and individuals, nurses, wards, hospitals and patients can be disciplined either informally or formally. This potential disciplinary mechanism reflects similar efforts to control the work of doctors in recent years by an array of accounting procedures and new agencies which have been promoted by the UK government (Traynor and Rafferty 1997, Traynor 2000).

What looks like poor implementation, Latimer suggests, is better described as active transformation – or 'translation' to use Latour's (1991) term – on the part of nurses who, like any presumed implementer of an innovation, transform a new technology in ways that help them to organize their work and enhance their own identity as professionals. This is not necessarily done in a fully conscious, programmatic way. However, the potential of the Nursing Process and other systems that enable accountability to affect the consciousness and activity of nurses is real because they bring to the fore issues of accountability, reward and reprimand. Nevertheless, any understanding of the uptake of the Nursing Process and similar accountability systems that does not include a sophisticated understanding of nurses as active in the process makes the mistake of seeing the operation of power in a simplistic and binary fashion: 'All these technologies supposedly enhance the visibility and accountability of practitioners, making their work more available to scrutiny in relation to particular standards or measures of performance' (Harraway 1985: 215). '[However] A diffusion model fails to reflect how actors do not simply implement, or fail to implement technologies, but rather deploy technologies, like any other artifact, as extensions (Strathern 1991) of themselves in their day-to-day organizing and identity work' (Latimer 1995: 216).

Both Purkis and Latimer go further than proposing that nurses are altered by the Nursing Process. They claim that patients too are caught up and transformed. As nurses are represented as problem identifiers and solution implementers, individual patients are presented as the source of a range of problems – some physical, some emotional, and all potentially amenable to nursing interventions. In Strathern's and in Latimer's words, the patients become 'extensions' of the nurses in their endeavours to represent themselves within a particular professional identity: '. . . behind the introduction of the Nursing Process is a notion that nurses can separate their understandings of patients from their day-to-day management of wards. The assumption is that they can "see" patients objectively and yet holistically' (Latimer 1995: 216).

Another consequence of understanding the implementation of the process from a translation rather than from a diffusion perspective is that it can explain the lack of consistency (which we noted above) in the way that the process is 'fabricated' by actors in different local settings or by educators or theorizers:

> Social actors (nurses, doctors, social workers, managers), then, can be considered not just as deploying particular products ('audit', 'Nursing Process', 'task-centred case management', 'problem-oriented records', RM systems) badly or well but as fabricating these 'technologies' locally and specifically as materials and devices to help produce further effects and institute particular relations.
>
> (Latimer 1995: 217)

Latimer makes two final points. First, compared to the established power base of medicine, nursing is in a more fragile position. While medicine has largely, or at least at the time she was writing, rejected taking up managerialist devices to demonstrate its value (e.g. in strident value-for-money terms), nursing has been preoccupied with its uncertain professional status and power base. This lack of confidence has led to its vulnerability to being drawn on to the ground of managerialism, or any other ground that looks likely to enhance its apparent effectiveness and value. Second, she questions the notion that 'there can be universal models of how nurses do (or should do) nursing' (Latimer 1995: 218). Certain elite groups within the nursing profession are concerned to promote 'stories of order', which can, they believe, enhance the ostensible rationality and value of the profession. The unforeseen consequence of such a project is that where nurses do not appear to conform, or live up to, these models they can be seen as failing in the implementation of valuable innovations. Nurses' apparent indifference to the evidence-based practice movement has been viewed in this way, while a similar scepticism in medicine was seen more positively even though the arguments that each group made were similar (Naylor 1995, McClarey and Duff 1997, Traynor 2002). To apply the translation approach to understanding 'deviations' from standard (or rather idealized) practice allows us to see a more favourable picture of nurses as competent and sophisticated social and political actors rather than failed implementers.

CONCLUSION

We believe that the promotion of the Nursing Process developed in two important contexts: one was the influence of medical discourse as seen in the move from the 'Yale' process to the 'Catholic' process. The second was a predominant belief in scientific and human progress. This evolutionary approach was applied as a way of understanding the uptake of scientific and technological innovations within nursing. As a supposedly formalizing endeavour, the evolutionary approach was seen to have the promise of rationalizing and unifying the diversity of nursing practice and nursing consciousness. In the specific context of managerialism, this approach could make explicit the contribution of nursing care to health outcomes and, hopefully, safeguard the profession in a time of financial stringency and insecurity. For many reasons, the process was locally 'fabricated', and also written about, in ways that did not give rise to any unified sense of what it actually was. It came to stand as an empty signifier for 'what nurses do' or for some idealized essence of nursing practice. Unfortunately, a combination of its association with a positive value for the profession, the bewildering variety of its embodiment and the widespread view that nurses were 'failing' to implement it has meant that, during its history, the process has produced some major negative effects on practitioners.

We suggest that a less totalizing (Lyotard 1979) and essentialist view, by which we mean, broadly, less concern for a quest for the discovery and expression of a single essence of nursing practice, contrary to what many nursing leaders have appeared to believe, could produce conditions more satisfying and less conflicting with everyday experience for the majority of practising nurses.

REFERENCES

Adorno T, Horkheimer A 1979 Dialectic of enlightenment. Verso, London
Beedholm K 2003 Forandring og træghed i den sygeplejefaglige diskurs. PhD

Copenhagen University, Copenhagen

Dingwall R, Allen D 2001 The implications of healthcare reforms for the profession of nursing. Nursing Inquiry 8(2): 64–74

Duldt BW 1995 Nursing Process. The science of nursing in the curriculum. Nurse Educator 20(1): 24–29

Fawcett J 1984 Analysis and evaluation of conceptual models of nursing. F A Davis, Philadelphia

Foucault M 1972 The archaeology of knowledge. Routledge, London

Foucault M 1977 Discipline and punish. Penguin, Harmondsworth

Foucault M 1980 The eye of power. In: Gordon C (ed.) Power/knowledge. Selected interviews and other writings 1972–1977. Harvester Wheatsheaf, Hemel Hempstead: 146–165

Foucault M 1984 What is enlightenment? In: Rabinow P (ed.) The Foucault reader. Penguin, Harmondsworth: 32–50

Foucault M 1991 Politics and the study of discourse In: Burchell G, Gordon C, Miller P (eds) The Foucault effect. Harvester Wheatsheaf, Hemel Hempstead

Harraway D 1985 A manifesto of cyborgs: science, technology and socialist feminism in the 1980s. Socialist Review 80: 65–107

Heath H 1998 Paradigm dialogues and dogma: finding a place for research, nursing models and reflective practice. Journal of Advanced Nursing 28(2): 288–294

Henderson V 1987 Nursing Process – a critique. Holistic Nursing Practice 1(3): 7–18

Hunter D 1994 From tribalism to corporatism: the managerial challenge to medical dominance In: Gabe J, Kelleher D, Williams G (eds) Challenging medicine. Routledge, London: 1–22

Laclau E, Mouffe C 1985 Hegemony and socialist strategy. towards a radical democratic politics. Verso, London

Lane V, Lawler J 2003 Pap smear brochures, misogyny and language: a discourse analysis and feminist critique. Nursing Inquiry 4(4): 262–267

Latimer J 1995 The Nursing Process re-examined: diffusion or translation? Journal of Advanced Nursing 22: 213–220

Latour B 1987 Science in action: how to follow scientists and engineers through society. Harvard University Press, Cambridge, MA

Latour B 1991 Technology is society made durable. In: Law J (ed.) A sociology of monsters: essays on power, technology and domination. Routledge, London: 103–131

Lyotard J-F 1979 The postmodern condition: a report on knowledge. Manchester University Press, Manchester

McClarey M, Duff M 1997 Clinical effectiveness and evidence-based practice. Nursing Standard 11(52): 33–35

McKenna H 1997 Nursing theories and models. Routledge, London

Meleis A 1985 Theoretical nursing: development and progress. J B Lippincott and Co., Philadelphia

Naylor C D 1995 Grey zones of clinical practice: some limits to evidence-based medicine. Lancet 346: 840–842

Nutting M, Dock 1907 A history of nursing: the evolution of nursing systems from the earliest times to the foundation of the first English and American training schools. G P Putnam's Sons, London

Pollitt C 1993 Managerialism and the public services. Blackwell, Oxford

Powers P 2002 A discourse analysis of nursing diagnosis. Qualitative Health Research 12(7): 945–965

Prentice S 1991 What will we find at the market? Health Visitor 65(1): 9–11

Purkis M E 1999 Embracing technology: an exploration of the effects of writing nursing. Nursing Inquiry 6(3): 147–156

Rogers E M 1985 Diffusion of innovations. The Free Press, New York

Strathern M 1991 Partial connections. Rowman and Littlefield, Lanham, MD

Traynor M 1999 Managerialism and nursing: beyond profession and oppression. Routledge, London

Traynor M 2000 Purity, Conversion and the evidence-based movements. Health: An Interdisciplinary Journal for the Social Study of Health, Illness and Medicine 4(2): 139–158

Traynor M 2002 The oil crisis, risk and evidence-based practice. Nursing Inquiry 9(3): 162–169

Traynor M A, Rafferty M 1997 The NHS R&D context for nursing research: a working paper. Centre for Policy in Nursing Research, London School of Hygiene & Tropical Medicine, London

University of Waterloo Ontario 2002 Themes in 19th century evolutionary theory. University of Waterloo Ontario Department of Anthropology. http://www.arts.uwaterloo.ca/ANTHRO/rwpark/courses/Anth352F02/anth352evolutionarytheory.html

Varcoe C 1996 Disparagement of the nursing process: the new dogma? Journal of Advanced Nursing 23(1): 120–125

Chapter **4**

The Nursing Process in UK mental health care: application to a field of nursing

Martin F. Ward

INTRODUCTION

The Nursing Process has been implemented in many fields or disciplines of nursing – general nursing, mental health nursing, community health nursing – to name but a few. In some of these areas, there was a better 'fit' between the field and the Nursing Process than in others. One such field with a good fit is mental health nursing. In this chapter, the implementation of the Nursing Process in the field of mental health nursing in one country (the UK) will be explored. This is a particularly interesting case study because, during the time of implementation, mental health nursing in the UK changed from being essentially hospital-based to having a large community-based component.

The following aspects of mental health nursing in the UK supported the implementation of the Nursing Process in this field of nursing.

- Nursing was beginning to shake off its reputation by the 1970s as being a medically subservient profession. Rigorous unidisciplinary research was being undertaken and senior practitioners were being educated to higher degree levels. There were moves to determine the roles and responsibilities of nursing through nurse-oriented frameworks, protocols and standards. In some fields of care, such actions created friction between nursing and the other professions because none of them were willing to change the existing status quo and, indeed, some of them saw a more autonomous and self-directing nursing workforce as offering a direct threat to the existing, well-established, power differentials. In mental health, there was less of a problem because the core disciplines (psychiatry, nursing, social work, psychology and, more latterly, occupational therapy) already had lower power thresholds and, to a certain degree, each had clinical responsibilities that overlapped and enabled some joint decision-making.
- To a certain degree, the Nursing Process demanded an element of autonomous practice from nurses if it was to be effective and, in a psychiatric setting, this was much more easily achievable. Patients spent most of their time in the company of nurses who invariably managed their own time, and did not have to link this with the demands of medical procedures or clinical routines. The period of time that mental health nurses spent in company with their patients was often greater than that of nurses in any other field. This, combined with the fact that they were not encumbered with large numbers of clinical procedures to carry out on their patients and that, in fact, their fundamental role was to use their interpersonal skills as their primary tool for intervention, enabled them to concentrate more closely on the organization of that care, its planning, implementation and evaluation.
- The process, as described by such writers as Marriner (1979) and Kron (1981), fitted well with the problem-based nature of mental health care, and offered its nursing practitioners a framework within which to develop not only their patient care but their own professional growth. The Nursing Process linked the ground-breaking work of nursing theorists, such as Abdullah (1957), Henderson (1960) and Peplau (1960), with the clinical environment in which it could be developed and enhanced.

The development, implementation and ongoing use of the Nursing Process, and its various derivative forms, within UK mental health nursing might be described in a number of ways: as a contest of wills between those nurses who wanted to change the way nurses work towards a more professional setting, and nurses and other health professionals who favoured the old models. The implementation of the Nursing Process can also be described as a waste of resources with little or no return for the effort. In the final instance, the implementation of the Nursing Process into UK mental health nursing practice in the 2000s can be described as a successful campaign in disguising the obvious, in which the essentials of the Nursing Process were implemented without calling them the Nursing Process. None of these descriptions, however, encompass the whole truth, but their usage can be understood when one examines what has actually taken place in mental health care in the UK since the late 1970s.

EARLY IMPLEMENTATION

At the time of the introduction of the Nursing Process to UK mental health services (nearly 25 years ago at the time of writing this chapter), psychiatry was still the dominant force amongst the core mental health professions. Nursing actions were mainly derived from decisions stemming from medical diagnosis, whilst in-patient services were still the predominant point of care delivery (King 1991).

Much of the early 1980s were spent considering a wide range of service changes within mental health. The Nursing Process, seen by many outside nursing and, to a certain degree, by many within it, was an extra commitment that rated low on the list of priorities. Why was this? For a start, many of the organizational changes hinged upon the necessity to restructure the whole operational activity of mental health care. The hospital closure programme had begun to take shape, and many established and traditional institutions were being aggressively encouraged by those who funded them to consider in-patient 'rationalization'. This meant developing community services to take over from the basic hospital set up and eventually selling of much of the estate that had housed the majority of mental health services. With this change came new roles for mental health nurses, including an increase in their roles in relation to both patient care and management (Butterworth et al 1986). It might be imagined that the introduction of the nursing process would be seen as an ideal way to enhance this activity but this was not to be the case. It has to be remembered that the Nursing Process was new to most practitioners. The disruption associated with massive organizational changes meant that few had the time to consider altering the whole way that they structured their care delivery actions. Certainly a variety of directives from the UK Department of Health meant that the process was kept in the professional eye but the strongest focus of service providers was the necessity to capitalize upon the financial gain of selling large areas of highly sought after land to developers.

Perhaps as a consequence of meeting the needs of nurses in their developing roles but more likely as a response to changes taking place in other parts of the world, the nursing profession itself was examined more closely with regard to their academic preparation, research activities and the actions of leaders and managers. The impact of this work had far more significance for the implementation of the Nursing Process. Papers began to appear in some profusion concerning various applications, in a variety of clinical locales and for differing conditions; much of this activity was based within a mental health setting (Stevenson 1984, Milne and Thurton 1986, Oliver and Redfern 1991). These included texts that outlined the nursing process as applied to psychiatry (Ward 1985, Meades 1989), different applications (Chapman 1988, Armitage 1989), patient involvement (Reynolds 1982, Richards and Lambert 1987, Shields and Morrison 1989) and, at last, papers that considered problem-solving activities associated with implementation of the Nursing Process (Shea 1986, Walton 1986, Mulhearn 1989, Ward 1989).

Implementing the Nursing Process was not as simple as saying 'Let's do it!' As the author and colleagues were to discover, a decade or so later when trying to implement evidence into practice, people do not accept change readily (Jackson et al 1999). The problem was not just a resistance to altering the way that things had been done for a long period of time and that practitioners simply did not want to interrupt the status quo, nor even that there was a lack of leadership on the part of nursing management, who, in the main, knew less about the Nursing Process than their staff. The major difficulty was that nursing, as it was carried out at this time, was not structured in a way that could readily adapt to accommodate advanced or specialized therapeutic nursing actions. One has to remember that, in nursing, the realization that in-patient services were giving way to community care was only just beginning and nurses had traditionally managed these institutional settings through a task-oriented approach to care. Thus, it was that each day was regimented by a series of routines and rituals with nursing actions taking precedence over patient needs. Hospitals, even to this day, tend to be run in support of hospital priorities: meals come when the kitchen sends them, not when the patient might be hungry; and medications are given at prescribed times and not necessarily at the best time for the individual patient. During the mid-1980s, mental health nurses, though being more flexible in their working actions than their general counterparts, managed patient care through actions that supported the hospital set-up. As such, the concept of individualized patient care was still to be developed as more than rhetoric and what mattered during the day was to 'get things done' rather than organizing care so that it corresponded with patient priorities. This is not to suggest that care was inadequate or that nurses did not care about their patients, it was simply that they had no understanding of different ways of doing what they had always done and, in most cases, been trained to do – keep the patients safe and attend to their basic needs.

The Nursing Process could not have been implemented into this rather rigid way of working without additional changes being made to the structure of nursing. These came in the form of the implementation of primary or team nursing, more effective reporting mechanisms, raising of nurses' awareness of their observational and assessment skills, and the development of a greater understanding of nursing models (or philosophical underpinnings to clinical care). These, linked with the advent (or, in many cases, the rediscovery) of clinical supervision, were to revolutionize the way that mental nursing was carried out and would provide the basis for operational changes that were radically to reshape the whole of mental health care within the UK.

For this to happen, however, nurses had to raise their general level of academia (education, research, evidence for practice) and give credence to the necessity to make more sense of their clinical actions. Carrying out fundamental activities of daily living, mixed with a basic understanding of psychiatry and combined with idiosyncratic personal approaches to the application of nursing theory in a hospital setting requires a great deal of time and effort. Ultimately, though, routinized and naïve approaches to care prohibit professional growth and suffocate those who seek to improve or develop themselves and the care they offer. Indeed, within a care setting with such rigid routine care, those who attempt to make changes are seen as radical and destabilizing. Observers of the Nursing Process at this time would have seen two distinct groups of individuals within mental health nursing: those who wanted to try new ways of working and who perceived in the Nursing Process the true nature of what the work should be, and those who represented the 'old school'. The latter group were adamant that things could not be done differently, and that, in fact, 'all this' had been tried before and it was damaging to the patients to keep messing them about simply to satisfy the demands of a small group of meddling revolutionaries. The truth was, perhaps, somewhere in the middle. Certainly, the disruption caused both to patient care in the early stages, and to traditional nursing administration, may well have had a detrimental effect on the overall quality of care, especially where so many resources were galvanized (and ultimately squandered) to resist its implementation. There is also no doubt that many experienced mental health nurses found themselves feeling de-skilled by the new approach. In addition, as is often the case when change does take place, many of these groups of practitioners left mental health nursing because they felt that they were devalued and were also unable to cope with the apparent complexity of what was being developed as an alternative to their experience. It is also true to say that not everything that was done in the name of the implementation of the Nursing Process was either appropriate or done for the reason of improving patient care alone. For instance, systems were developed around the process, which were designed primarily to operationalize managerial changes and had little to do with patient care. The view that the Nursing Process was the panacea to mend all the ills of mental health nursing certainly did exist in some during that time, and there is no doubt that it damaged the reputation of the process and made its implementation a much more difficult task.

Conversely, it is also true that nursing could not have continued in the way that it had done to this point, nor could it have achieved the status of an autonomous professional group within the core psychiatric disciplines, without the aid of improved systems of working, effective decision-making models, a complete overhaul of its internal administration, its adoption of a higher academic preparation and the development of roles that enabled all of the above to become active.

EDUCATIONAL CHANGES

Mental health nursing in the UK has always attempted to establish itself as an autonomous group within the nursing family (Nolan 1993). Way back in 1920 mental health nurses had been accorded a supplementary register of qualified nurses by the General Nursing Council of the UK, with their own final examination and their own training programme, but with a single entry portal into the nursing system. In the early 1990s, this uniqueness was, to a certain degree, taken away from them with the advent of new educational developments. Yet, paradoxically, it was these same developments that enabled mental health nurses to achieve a level of professional maturity that they had not had previously whilst also giving them a framework in which to implement the Nursing Process effectively. Thus, it was that, during this period of time, the Nursing Process and mental health nursing professionalism were intertwined, with one acting as the catalyst for the other.

The new approaches to education were the result of the then UK governing body for nurses, the UK Council for Nursing and Midwifery (UKCC), shifting emphasis from traditional nurse training to nurse education, raising the basic level of entry into nursing from certificate to diploma level and placing the educational centre within universities, as opposed to separate centres, usually located within hospitals. This programme, known as Project 2000, had a syllabus based around the components of the process and so demanded that students had to explore it in some detail whilst clinical areas had to be using it to have students placed with them (Hollingworth 1986). Project 2000 led to the official recognition of the Nursing Process as the method by which mental health nursing should be undertaken, and demanded that mental health nursing students had to undergo an 18-month period of common educational preparation with their general nursing colleagues before moving to the final 18 months of specialist mental health nursing. In one stroke, mental health nurses developed a more systematic approach to their work, being able to demonstrate both what they were doing and how they were doing it, yet they lost ground in their attempts to be seen as significantly different from their general nursing counterparts.

THE EARLY 1990s: A PERIOD OF CONSOLIDATION

We arrive in the 1990s with mental health nurses both gaining and losing ground in terms of their own professional identity, but certainly maintaining a degree of momentum in terms of their actual ability to deliver individualized nursing care. They came to the 1990s in much better shape to deal with the policy changes that were soon to be enacted than they had been at the start of the decade before. As is often the case with policy change, however, it does not take account of the predicaments of specific groups. Nursing, despite its practitioners being better prepared, still had not consolidated its developments, new ideas and approaches to care delivery and its organization (Salvage 1990).

It is also worth noting that, at the same time as the key changes and reforms in mental health service provision were taking place, the term

'Nursing Process', began to drop out of common usage. The author carried out a piece of research during this time that explored the implementation of the process within a psychiatric context across several health providers (Ward 1991). What was obvious was the term itself meant nothing to patients or their carers. It had not, as such, transferred itself from a nursing term to one which had meaning for the wider social community, unlike terms of medicine, social work or psychology. In addition, the sociolinguistics of nursing itself meant that very few of the other core psychiatric disciplines had any real understanding of what was meant by the term. What they understood were the actions of nurses within a multidisciplinary context and in support of team care provision. It was probably this recognition of separate clinical responsibilities that enabled the Nursing Process to continue to have impact upon the work of nurses whilst also itself, apparently, disappearing from having any effective role to play.

During this time, however, one of the key benefits from Nursing Process usage was an increase in the communication that was undertaken by nurses with other professional groups on the part of patients (Salvage 1990, Ward 1992). Certainly this corresponded with developments that were beginning to have impact throughout the whole of the psychiatric community; the introduction of genuine multidisciplinary working practices and developing roles within community settings for mental health nurses.

The hospital closure programme, which had seen a major overhaul of point of delivery services generally in mental health, was at its height at this time and, as a consequence, nurses were being offered the opportunity to develop their own practice in areas where other core psychiatric disciplines had little or no involvement. A series of other government-led initiatives were driving mental health care during this period and it was perhaps these, rather than any perceived efficacy associated with Nursing Process application, that brought enduring and sustained changes within the roles and responsibilities of nursing. The major reforms of the National Health Service focused in mental health on community care, patient involvement and quality assurance.

In 1991, the government launched The Patients Charter (Department of Health 1991a). Implicit within this was the directive that each patient should have assigned to them a named nurse who would take responsibility for managing their care. The named nurse would have a group of patients and would be supported by associate nurses who would act on the patients' behalf in the absence of the named nurse. This reform was pushed through very rapidly, partly owing to nurse managers responding to pressure from the Department of Health and partly because of user groups demanding its implementation. Just over a year later, Wright (1993) reported that the named nurse had been implemented within all nursing specialties and, whilst there was some scepticism within mental health nursing circles as to the motivation for such haste, it was evident that, within the specialty, named nursing was readily adopted. Interestingly enough, it was not the concept of the named nurse that caused problems but that of the associate nurse. There were serious concerns about who these associate nurses should be and who should support student nurses in this system. It was not until the mid-1990s that these problems were comprehensively addressed (Dargen 1997).

What must be obvious to the reader, as indeed it was to many nurse commentators at the time, was that this was no more than the application of primary nursing in another guise. As such, those that had already adopted such an approach in conjunction with the Nursing Process found very little difficulty shifting to either the new title or the use of the approach. The fundamental difference was that, whereas the introduction of primary nursing had been an informal response on the part of practitioners and nurse educationalists to a management problem associated with the performance of the Nursing Process, the named nurse was mandatory across all forms of health care. By redefining primary nursing as an obligatory component of patient care, the UK government had ensured that the organizational setting for the Nursing Process was in place. As mental health progressed to a more varied and sophisticated service, it also meant that its nurses were better able to shoulder responsibility for individual as well as individualized case loads.

These issues were further enhanced as the decade progressed. Key workers, who had to take primary responsibility for the patient and be identified to the patient, were introduced into community mental health practice with similar roles as named nurses, but allowing for the key worker to belong to a range of health professions, whilst the Care Programme Approach (CPA), a system of planned discharge and support for patients either discharged from in-patient care or admitted directly into community care, used the system to maintain care management (Department of Health 1991b). In this way, planning of care, a concept fundamental to the Nursing Process, was institutionalized.

In 1993, the Department of Health in England published a policy guidance document called 'A vision for the future: the nursing, midwifery and health visiting contribution to health and health care' (Department of Health 1993). One of the five named key areas in the report was concerned with research and supervision and, in particular, one of 12 key targets to be addressed was specifically related to clinical supervision. Although such approaches to professional support had been long standing within psychotherapy and social work, they were, as Hill (1989) points out, relatively unknown within mental health nursing up until the latter stages of the 1980s. Clinical supervision was defined in this document as: 'a formal process of professional support and learning which enables individual practitioners to develop knowledge and competence, assume responsibility for their own practice and enhance consumer protection and safety in complex situations' (Department of Health 1993).

This approach to nurse support and development, later refined by authors such as Butterworth et al (1996) and Cutcliffe (1997), combined with a national review of mental health nursing (Department of Health 1994), supported clinical supervision through a systematic approach that very much reflected Nursing Process methodology, and allowed the development of the skills and knowledge mental health nurses needed to realize the Nursing Process fully in this area of nursing.

As community mental health began to take shape, with some inevitable organizational problems, attention was drawn towards the need to keep the public safe from the so-called dangerous mentally ill. This led to a certain amount of tension developing between those who were responsible for managing care and those whose duty was social order and public safety. The consequence of this tension was a gradual but insidious expansion of tools designed to evaluate both perceived and potential risk of harm to the general public, and the need to reduce suicidal behaviours within in-patient settings. In official enquiries, 20% of suicides are regarded as preventable (Standing Nursing and Midwifery Advisory Committee 1999), and around a quarter of suicides occur in the UK within 3 months of discharge from in-patient care (Department of Health 2002). To a certain degree, mental health care within the UK became overburdened with the need to undertake this work and nursing was, and remains, the lead professional discipline for carrying out these assessments (O'Rourke et al 1997). A nursing shortage, the reduction in in-patient facilities and, at that time, the absence of a coherent community care strategy, placed even greater strains on the nursing profession. One of the effects of this for the Nursing Process was the necessity for nurses to place greater emphasis on procedures and patterns of work and, in particular, assessments based on standardized forms. This removed a certain amount of the flexibility associated with process assessments and focused attention away from a more holistic interpretation of individual patient needs. Perhaps more significantly it also meant that care was often directed specifically at special observations which restricted the overall care available to patients and was unpopular with many of them (Jones et al 2000). A series of high-profile audits of in-patient services indicated serious problems with care provision, and pointed to an absence of care continuity, one of the basic outcomes of good Nursing Process usage.

At the same time, there were considerable changes taking place within forensic mental health with a dramatic increase in the number of nurses involved in all levels of secure care. In this type of care setting, risk was of paramount importance and standardized assessments and long-term care planning inhibited a creative use of the Nursing Process. In particular, forensic nurses had been unable to develop objectives for care processes because these were restricted by the fact that the patient was unlikely to be discharged and/or rehabilitated for a very long time. In consequence monotoned, single-dimensional care packages had been produced. Forensic nurses found it easy to undertake the paperwork for the Nursing Process but more difficult to make that paperwork meaningful in terms of patient care.

Community care also was undergoing massive change. The Nursing Process has always been more difficult to implement within a community setting (Ward 1992). It has to be recognized that many community nurses simply did not plan their care in relation to other care providers. There may be many reasons why community and hospital nurses did not work well together, and many of them relate to the organizational structures in which they work. It was also found, however, that the situation was exacerbated by an absence of care planning and, in particular, effective discharge planning (Llovera et al 2003). The result was that community and in-patient care became polemic services, separated both geographically as well as organizationally. The government responded to this polarization by introducing, first, case management (Ward et al 1999, Ward and Stuart 2004) and, later, assertive outreach and home treatments (Addis and Gamble 2004). Case management placed greater emphasis upon the ability of individual workers to plan effective interventions with and on behalf of the patient (Anthony and Crawford 2000), while assertive outreach and home treatments enhanced the community care of clients who were difficult to engage.

There remains one aspect of reform and development that has yet to be described, and it is perhaps this, more than anything else, that will sustain the Nursing Process within a mental health setting. Care pathways, beloved by some, abhorred by others, have been developed during the 1990s and more latterly in the early 2000s to safeguard the planned nature of a patient's care. Jones (2003: 670) describes care pathways as '. . . a paper based format, which details the expected problems, interventions and outcomes for a specified disorder'. In reality, they deal with a condition rather than a person, but are usually designed in such a way as to take into account individualized problems and to deal with the uniqueness of a person's response to his or her own illness. In some ways, they could be regarded as the same as the Nursing Process' standard care plans except that they tend to be more multiprofessional in nature. Care pathways have become very popular within mental health, as mental health practitioners struggle to prove the clinical efficacy of interventions and to maintain health outcomes according to government targets. Inherent within the process of developing these pathways is a system akin to that of developing clinical guidelines. Thus, evidence is used to prescribe the best ways of working in relation to different problems. Again, it is predominantly nurses that use the pathways to underscore the interventions that they need to employ to deal effectively with a person's problems. Also, whilst the care pathways cannot be equated to the Nursing Process, both are methods of problem-solving, they both demand the same components of decision-making and they both require intensive evaluation against patient baselines to be able to function properly. It could be argued, therefore, that the next generation of Nursing Process actions has arrived in the guise of care pathways.

During the 1990s, therefore, the Nursing Process was subsumed by operational reforms, many of which involved the same concepts and principles espoused by the Nursing Process. As such, the Nursing Process was lost to the nursing vocabulary in the UK, even while in effect being used in practice.

CONCLUSION

We should not assume that the process itself has actually disappeared, despite what the reader of this chapter may think. The Nursing Process is still taught within the educational preparation of student nurses, although now it tends to have been assimilated into the process of describing care practices rather than being a separate entity in its own right. Nurses in mental health care use process actions on a daily basis, especially within in-patient setting and in conjunction with named nurse and primary nursing systems. In the community, CPA, key workers, case management, assertive outreach and home treatments have utilized the process to ensure that nurses, the main providers of community mental health care, are in a position to observe, assess, plan, deliver and assess appropriate interventions.

In the long run, care pathways will provide a measure of stability to care which can otherwise often be fragmented and uncoordinated.

The final question has to be, has anything changed from where this chapter began? Is there still a *contest of wills* between those who want to implement change and those who do not? The answer is probably no, since the main battle for the Nursing Process was fought several decades ago. Has there been *little return for all the effort*? Mental health nursing has come a long way in three decades, mostly without the aid of research or evidence, and mostly on the back of policy, yet it has come a long way. The nursing process provided nurses with the rubric upon which most, if not all, of this change could be based, so the author would suggest that the effort was worth it. And finally, has the *obvious been disguised?* Undoubtedly, yes! There are still those who will tell you that nursing does not use the process any more, despite the fact they use both its components and principles on a daily basis without realizing it.

REFERENCES

Abdullah F 1957 Methods of establishing covert aspects of nursing problems. Nursing Research 6(1): 4–23

Addis J, Gamble C 2004 Assertive outreach nurse's experience of engagement. Journal of Psychiatric and Mental Health Nursing 11: 452–460

Anthony P, Crawford P 2000 Service user involvement in care planning: the mental health nurse's perspective. Journal of Psychiatric and Mental Health Nursing 7(5): 425–434

Armitage P 1989 Primary nursing in long term psychiatric care. Senior Nurse 9(9): 22–24

Butterworth T, Bishop V, Carson J 1996 First steps towards evaluating clinical supervision in nursing and health visiting. 1. Theory, policy and practice development. A review. Journal of Clinical Nursing 5(2): 127–132

Chapman G E 1988 Reporting therapeutic discourse in a therapeutic community. Journal of Advanced Nursing 13(2): 255–264

Cutcliffe J 1997 Evaluating the success of clinical supervision. British Journal of Nursing 6(13): 725

Dargan R 1997 The Named nurse in practice. Baillière Tindell, London

Department of Health 1991a The patient's charter. HMSO, London

Department of Health 1991b The care programme approach for people with a mental illness, referred to specialist psychiatric services. HC(90)23/LASSL(90)11 Joint Health and Social Services Circular. HMSO, London

Department of Health 1993 A vision for the future: the nursing, midwifery and health visiting contribution to health and health care. HMSO, London

Department of Health 1994 Working in partnership: a collaborative approach to care. Report of the Mental Health Nursing Review Team. HMSO, London

Department of Health 2002 Mental health policy implementation guide: adult acute inpatient care provision. HMSO, London

Henderson V 1960 The nature of nursing. Macmillan, New York

Hargreaves I 1979 Theoretical considerations. In: Kratz C (ed.) The nursing process. Baillière Tindall, London

Hill J 1989 Supervision in the caring professions: a literature review. Community Psychiatric Nursing Journal 9(5): 9–15

Hollingworth S 1986 The nursing process: Implications for curriculum planning. Journal of Advanced Nursing 11: 211–216

Jackson A, Ward M F, Cutliffe J, Titchen A, Cannon B 1999 Practice development in mental health nursing, Part 11. Mental Health Nursing 2: 20–25

Jones A 2003 Perceptions on the development of a care pathway for people diagnosed with schizophrenia on acute psychiatric units. Journal of Psychiatric and Mental Health Nursing 10: 669–677

Jones J, Ward M F, Wellman N, Hall J, Lowe T 2000 Psychiatric in-patients' experience of nursing observation. Journal of Psychosocial Nursing and Health Services 38(12): 10–20

King D 1991 Moving on: from mental hospital to community care. Nuffield Hospitals Provincial Trust, Exeter

Kron T 1981 The management of patient care: putting leadership skills into practice, 5th edn. Saunders, Philadelphia

Llovera I, Ward M F, Ryan JG, LaTouche T, Sama A 2003 A survey of the emergency department population and their interest in preventive health education. Academic Emergency Medicine 10(2): 155–160

Marriner A (ed.) 1979 The nursing process: a scientific approach to care. Mosby, St Louis

Meades S 1989 Integrative care planning in acute psychiatry. Journal of Advanced Nursing 14: 630–639

Milne D, Thurton N 1986 Making the nursing process work in mental health. Senior Nurse 5(5): 33–34

Mulhearn S 1989 The nursing process: improving psychiatric admission assessment. Journal of Advanced Nursing 14: 808–814

Nolan P 1993 A history of mental health nursing. Chapman & Hall, London

Oliver S, Redfern S J 1991 Interpersonal communication between nurses and elderly patients: refinement of an observational tool. Journal of Advanced Nursing 16: 30–38

O'Rourke M M, Hammond S M, Davies E J 1997 Risk assessment and risk management: the way forward. Psychiatric Care 4(3): 104–106

Peplau H E 1960 Talking with patients. American Journal of Nursing 60: 964–966

Reynolds W 1982 Patient centred teaching: a further role for the psychiatric nurse teacher. Journal of Advanced Nursing 7: 469–475

Richards D A, Lambert P 1987 The nursing process: the effects on patient satisfaction with nursing care. Journal of Advanced Nursing 12(5): 559–562

Salvage J 1990 The theory and practice of the 'new nursing'. Nursing Times 86(4): 42–45

Shea H L 1986 A conceptual framework to study the use of the nursing care plan. International Journal of Nursing Studies 23(2): 147–157

Shields P J, Morrison P 1989 Consumer satisfaction on a psychiatric ward. Journal of Advanced Nursing 13: 396–400

Standing Nursing and Midwifery Advisory Committee 1999 Mental health nursing: addressing acute concerns. HMSO, London

Stevenson M 1984 Problems remain: trying to implement the nursing process in an acute area of psychiatry. Nursing Mirror 158: 1 Mental Health Forum V–V11

Walton J 1986 The nursing process in perspective. Department of Social Policy and Social Work, University of York, York

Ward M F 1985 The nursing process in psychiatry. Churchill Livingstone, Edinburgh

Ward M F 1989 Expressive objectives. Nursing Times 85(51): 61–63

Ward M F 1991 The effects of nursing process implementation within a psychiatric nursing context. Unpublished M.Phil. thesis. University of East Anglia, Norwich

Ward M F 1992 The nursing process in psychiatry, 2nd edn. Churchill Livingstone, Edinburgh

Ward M F, Stuart G 2004 Case management: perspectives of the United Kingdom and US system. In: Harrison M, Mitchell D (eds) Current issues in acute mental health nursing. Sage, London

Ward M F, Armstrong C, Lelliott P, Davies M 1999 Training, skills and caseload of community mental health workers involved in case management: an evaluation from the initial United Kingdom demonstration sites. Journal of Psychiatric and Mental Health Nursing 6(3): 187–198

Wright S 1993 The named nurse, midwife and health visitor – principles and practice. In Wright S (ed.) The named nurse, midwife and health visitor. National Health Service Management Executive, Leeds

Chapter 5

The Nursing Process and information technology

Elske Ammenwerth

INTRODUCTION

Nursing documentation is an important part of clinical documentation. A thorough nursing documentation system is usually seen as a precondition for good patient care, and for efficient communication and cooperation within the health professional team (Leiner and Haux 1996). Paper-based documentation systems have been introduced to support the Nursing Process documentation. Frequently, however, large amounts of poor-quality documentation and limited acceptance of the Nursing Process are reported, as also discussed by Davis et al (1994).

There have been many attempts to support the Nursing Process using computer-based documentation systems since the 1980s. Early examples include Romano et al (1982) and Lichten and Soble (1984). Typical aims are to reduce the documentation workload, increase the documentation quality and allow data to be reused for nursing management, nursing control and nursing research. Additional aims may be to increase the professionalization of nursing care and to support the implementation of the Nursing Process.

Despite considerable investment of both time and money, problems associated with computer-based documentation systems are frequently reported. Insufficient reflection of the complexity of the Nursing Process, lack of a standardized nursing terminology, computer-anxious users, fear of less individual care and too much control, high implementation and operation costs, and unclear benefits have all been identified in this regard (e.g. Harris 1990, Goossen et al 1997, Büssing and Herbig 1998).

Interest in the actual effects of computer-based nursing documentation systems have grown in the last years. Several studies have been conducted so far to evaluate the effects of information technology (IT) in nursing. These studies focus on various IT applications in nursing (e.g. patient monitoring vs. care planning) being installed in different environments (e.g. intensive care unit vs. normal wards) and being based on different technologies (e.g. stationary vs. mobile computers).

In this chapter, we will concentrate on revealing IT support for the documentation of the Nursing Process as the most challenging part of IT in nursing today. The aims of this chapter are to give an overview of IT applications in nursing in hospital settings and to discuss the effects of IT-based nursing plans.

IT IN NURSING: RECENT AND FUTURE DEVELOPMENTS

Information technology was introduced into hospitals in the 1960s and 1970s, the first systems being used in laboratories and administration. IT in nursing started in the early 1980s. A rough Medline overview based on the words 'computer', 'nursing' and 'documentation' finds about four papers before 1980, seven during 1981–1985, 22 for 1986–1990, 52 for 1991–1995 and 74 papers since 1996. At first, the focus of such papers was mostly on the introduction and evaluation of nursing documentation systems, later shifting to the use of nursing terminology within IT systems, IT in nursing education, IT to increase patient safety, and nursing informatics in general.

Applications of IT in nursing

Information technology in nursing in general can comprise different application components, which each support different tasks undertaken by nurses. We will now briefly discuss the typical application components that can be found on a hospital unit (ward). A more detailed overview can be found, for example, in Hannah et al (1999) or Saba (1997).

Nursing documentation

Components for nursing documentation typically comprise the complete support of all phases of the Nursing Process, from nursing assessment to nursing evaluation. Nursing anamnesis (i.e. the analysis and documentation of relevant information on previous and recent illnesses of the patient by the nurse) is usually supported by the ability to define and use individual forms (e.g. for social anamnesis), containing structured and unstructured information. Based on the information gathered in the assessment phase, a nursing care plan for an individual patient can then be created. To support this, typical nursing problems, aims and tasks can be predefined and selected during the creation of the care plan. Typical combinations of problems, aims and tasks can be combined in predefined or standard nursing care plans. After selecting suitable care plans, these predefined items and standards can be selected and adapted to the patient's individual needs. Mostly, items are removed (e.g. problems which do not apply). Sometimes, items are added (e.g. individual patient resources). A nurse using a predefined care plan must be encouraged to add individual patient resources and to eliminate the problems (and aims and tasks) which do not apply.

After care planning, the execution of planned tasks can be scheduled, if necessary. Based on this care plan, nursing tasks are executed and documented, usually using a time axis within the documentation form. The system allows the documentation of planned tasks or other tasks along with information of special observations or occurrences. In addition, nursing aims can be planned, checked and documented. Finally, nursing reports can be written. The description shows that the use of predefined care plans integrates the several steps of the Nursing Process (definition of problems and patient resources; derivation of nursing aims; planning of nursing tasks; evaluation of the process) into one care planning step (i.e. choosing and editing a patient-related care plan). This procedure appears to simplify care planning and may improve nurses' attitudes towards the Nursing Process. This makes care planning much easier and more efficient than is conventionally possible.

The predefined care plans used in computer-based components are usually based on a specific nursing terminology or nursing classification. Typically, the components are flexible enough to be able to support any possible terminological approach a hospital may want. For example, Büssing and Herbig (1998) present in detail the architecture of software that allows the reflection of different nursing models, such as Roper, Orem, Juchli or Krowinkel. This flexibility also means that many components are just a kind of shell, which must be filled with adequate content and structures in order to be used in a sensible way in daily practice.

This typical functionality of applications for nursing documentation supports the core phases of the Nursing Process. In addition, computer-based documentation systems usually offer functions for the management of predefined care plans, for utilizing nursing knowledge (such as nursing standards), for nursing management (e.g. documentation of nursing costs, ward-related statistics), and for the definition and use of predefined forms for special documentation purposes (e.g. wound documentation).

Other parts of the patient record, such as the so-called Cardex (the temperature chart together with medications and medical orders), are often not yet fully supported by computer-based components owing to the complexity of this interprofessionally used medium. Thus, full support of the Cardex together with the Nursing Process documentation is necessary to avoid several systems being used while documenting the care of one patient. However, an integrated information processing is usually preferred.

Patient management

Components for patient management enable nurses to conduct the administrative admission of a patient. Here nurses must be able to document at least the most important details for a patient, and to create a patient identification number and a case identification number. In addition, changes to patient data, as well as transfer and discharge details for patients may also be supported.

Order management

These application components support nurses in ordering special patient-related services, such as laboratory, pathology or radiology. In addition, the applications may support the retransmission of the results of an examination. These application components typically offer up-to-date catalogues of services on offer, as well as the possibility to copy patient data from the patient management component. Retransmitted results may be printed and/or included in the electronic patient record of the patient. Besides patient-related ordering, these components may also support ordering of general items, such as drugs and meals.

Ward management

Ward management comprises the distribution of patients to rooms and beds. Those components obtain or transfer patient data from the patient management component.

Staff planning

These components support planning of working times of the nurses on a ward. They are usually connected to components of general staff management and support planning by automatic decision-support functions.

State-of-the-art and vision for the future

Today, nearly all hospitals have IT support in the area of patient administration. Many already support staff planning, ward management and parts of nursing documentation. Only a minority of hospitals in Europe offer a complete computer-based support of all nursing tasks, including nursing documentation and Cardex.

The number of application components installed in a ward determines the technical equipment needed. Application components for patient administration and ward management can be supported by a sufficient number of stationary computers (installed, for example, in the ward office) but, for extensive nursing documentation, additional bedside terminals or mobile computers will be needed.

It can be expected in the future that the majority of nurses' tasks will be supported by IT, leading to comprehensive electronic patient record systems, which comprise most of the patient-related data. Nursing-related data will be one important part. However, this vision requires a significant investment in technology, comprising adequate numbers of stationary computers, bedside computers, mobile computers and a wireless Local Area Network (LAN). Mobile computers will be very important in the future, as nurses are typically rather mobile in their daily work. Such mobility from one work setting to another during a single working period is not well supported by the traditional stationary workstation.

EFFECTS OF IT-BASED NURSING PLANS ON NURSING CARE

The introduction of IT to support nursing care planning and nursing documentation has a number of effects on nursing care. In this section, we will take a closer look at the effects of IT on nursing. We will consider the following aspects: efficiency of nursing, quality of nursing documentation, professionalization of nursing care, and user acceptance issues. The analysis of the effects of IT-based nursing care planning will be based on a discussion of the available literature as well as on the results of the author's own studies in recent years.

IT and the efficiency of nursing

The introduction of IT often aims at increasing the efficiency of nursing care. For example, Bürkle et al (1999) found that about 30% of a nurse's time is needed for administrative and documentation purposes. This time may be reduced by computer-based nursing documentation, allowing more time for direct patient care.

Research shows that such time savings are indeed possible. For example, Allan and Englebright (2000) found a 55% decrease in charting time per patient 3 months after the implementation of a computerized documentation system on four medical–surgical units. In general, such a large reduction in charting time is mostly achieved through the use of predefined standardized care plans. The more homogeneous the treatment of the patients is, the better it can be covered by standardized care plans, the fewer adaptations the nurses have to do during individual care planning, leading to a significant decrease in time for care planning.

Other studies support this. Ammenwerth et al (2001), in a randomized study on one ward, found a decrease in the overall time needed for care planning from 43.3 minutes/patient to 16.4 minutes/patient in the first 3 months after implementation of computerized care planning. Harris (1990) estimated that the time for care planning might be no more than 3–5 minutes/patient after extended use of a computerized system. Van Gennip et al (1995) estimated that about 20 minutes were saved in the production of care planning shortly after the introduction of a nursing documentation system on three non-intensive care unit (ICU) wards.

However, those time savings will not occur when complete care planning has not been done before IT implementation. In this case, the time to develop a complete care plan will certainly rise compared to that before IT implementation, despite – or because of – the computer. Van Gennip et al (1995) found this effect on one ward where the overall documentation time rose after implementation. However, this greater time may be balanced by much more complete and higher quality nursing documentation.

Documentation of nursing interventions may similarly take more time. For example, Ammenwerth et al (2001) found that the time for documentation of tasks and for report writing more than doubled: from 2.0 to 4.8 minutes/patient per day for task documentation, and from 4.6 to 6.6 minutes/patient per day for report writing. This increase was explained by the much more detailed documentation of tasks after the introduction of IT, and by the initial problems for many nurses in using the keyboard for writing free-text reports.

Thus, it is not surprising that the literature shows somewhat mixed or inconclusive evidence with regard to overall time savings after the introduction of a nursing documentation system. For example, van Gennip et al (1995) found no change in the overall time needed for administration and communication, including documentation (which was between 35% and 50% of the overall nursing time), on three wards after the introduction of IT.

Even when the effort involved in producing nursing documentation is reduced, it is questionable whether the patient benefits from the time that may be saved by computers. We will present details of two major studies to show the mixed evidence. Pabst et al (1996) found a decrease in the time needed for documentation activities from 13.7% to 9.1% in a work sampling study before, and 3 months after, the implementation of comprehensive bedside nursing documentation system on one ward. The time for direct patient care rose from 31.9% before the implementation to 37.6% after 6 months. The time devoted to documentation decreased from 13.7% to 9.1%. Thus, he found that, after implementation, more time was spent with the patient.

In contrast, Pryor (1989), in a work-sampling study after the introduction of bedside terminals for nursing documentation on a ward before and 1 year after the introduction of a computerized nursing charting system, found a decrease in general paperwork from 24% to 16.9%, combined with an increase in computer use from 2.2% to 13.5%, and a decrease in direct patient care time from 32.5% to 27.3%. Thus, he found more negative than positive effects.

Besides their effect on nurses' time, computers may also affect communication. For example, Büssing and Herbig (1998) argue that a comprehensive electronic patient record may reduce the need for extensive oral communication sessions (e.g. during shift changes), and may lead to a disappearance of more informal forms of communication. Büssing and Herbig (1998) were critical with regard to this development.

Health care professionals may be in favour of computerized documentation, given that they have easy access to it, since computerized records improve availability (compared to paper records), completeness and especially legibility. In the study by Ammenwerth et al (2001), four physicians on a ward with computer-based nursing documentation were asked their opinions. They used the system mainly to read the nursing reports, which they now found much more readable than before. They usually did not look into the details of care planning and nursing documentation. They stated that, in general, they now accessed nursing documentation more often, and found the documentation transparency much better and its quality higher. Overall, all four physicians voted in favour of the new system.

A final remark should be made about the computer equipment on a ward. Many studies do not explain in detail how many computers have been introduced and where they have been located. The supply of adequate levels of computer equipment is the necessary precondition for computerized nursing documentation to be feasible and really helpful. For example, Newton (1995) found negative attitude of nurses with regard to a computer-based system. He argued that in this case, better equipment (e.g. an increase in number of terminals and the provision of mobile computers) would reduce the problems and improve the attitudes. Ammenwerth et al (2002) also found in a qualitative evaluation study of the introduction of a nursing documentation system that insufficient levels of equipment was one reason for low user acceptance and problems in the beginning on one ward. On this ward, only two stationary computers had been installed in the ward (duty) room, which was insufficient, as the nurses needed access to the documentation at the bedside as well. The missing information at the patient's bedside disturbed the usual nursing workflow. They compensated for this gap by reintroducing paper-based documentation as an intermediate, which led to duplicate documentation, increased time producing documentation and low user acceptance. An increase in the number of computers and a reorganization of documentation processes later increased user acceptance on this ward.

It is, however, interesting to note that even completely equipping a ward with bedside terminals may not be the best solution, as Pabst et al (1996) found in their study. Nurses in this study did not take the opportunity to record patient progress information directly at the bedside, mostly because they were put off by patients or their family. Thus, the technical equipment should be carefully planned beforehand, and planning should take into account not only the number of users and the places where documentation is carried out, but also the organizational environment of a ward and the users' opinions.

In conclusion, computer-based nursing documentation and especially care planning can reduce the time taken for documentation, and may even lead to more time for the patient. These benefits may, however, only occur after a long implementation period and depend heavily on the available technical equipment, which must match the needs of a given ward. Finally, the improved availability of information may also affect communication patterns within the health care team.

IT and the quality of nursing documentation

Computer-based nursing documentation can have an enormous impact on the quality of nursing documentation. Aspects that may be improved are clarity, completeness and the amount of documentation. Many studies confirm this. For example, van Gennip et al (1995) found in the evaluation of nursing documentation on three non-ICU wards in three hospitals that information was more complete, more readable and clearer. Kahl et al (1991) reported more complete, timely, readable and correct documentation after the introduction of bedside terminals to a nursing documentation system on two wards. A detailed evaluation of the completeness of documentation after introduction of a nursing information system with care planning was also performed by Larrabee (2001) in a 100-bed hospital. Within the first 6 months after implementation, he did not find an improvement of completeness. However, after retraining of the users, the completeness of the documentation of both nursing assessment and intervention improved.

Another comprehensive evaluation was carried out by Newton (1995), who found, 3 months after the introduction of computer-based care planning on 16 wards, an increase in completeness and quality of documentation, measured with a standardized instrument. For example, more patients now had an assessment or a care plan, the problem list was more complete and more goals were evaluated than without the computer. A comparable increase in quality of documentation, as judged by the Joint Commission for Accreditation for Healthcare Organization (JCAHO) standards, was also found by McBride and Nagle (1996). Pabst et al (1996) even found that nurses using a comprehensive nursing documentation system updated the care plans more often.

Not all studies, however, found only positive effects for IT systems. For example, Pryor (1989) found an increase in completeness and consistency 1 year after the introduction of a bedside computerized nursing charting system, but also a drop in currency of the care plans from 70% to 43%. Büssing and Herbig (1998) argued that IT-based care planning might become a purely mechanical selection process when using the computer. Ammenwerth et al (2001) found in a direct comparison of 30 computer-based and 30 paper-based sets of documentation on one psychiatric ward, shortly after the introduction of a computer-based documentation system, both improvements and deteriorations in quality. On one hand, the completeness of documentation rose. For example, 79% of the patients with computer-based documentation now had a complete care plan (compared to 50% of the other patients). The average number of problems, aims and tasks had increased by between 100% and 400%. The legibility was 100% vs. 14%. In the computer-based groups, however, several severe quality problems were identified. For example, care plans were often unspecific and too long. Many tasks had been planned but were never executed. Overall, the quality of the documentation in both groups was judged as nearly equal (2.3 and 2.4 on a 5-point Likert scale) by two external reviewers.

This study was reproduced and extended in a subsequent study on four wards (two somatic and two psychiatric wards) by Mahler et al (2002) and Mahler et al (2005). In these studies, 20 records from each ward were analysed at three different times: before the introduction of the system, about 3 months after the implementation and again about 9–20 months after the implementation. Altogether, 240 documentations were analysed, based on a quantitative and qualitative checklist, by two external nursing experts. After the implementation of the computer-based documentation system, the nursing documentation became more complete. For example, on the two somatic wards, no care planning was done at the first measurement. At the third measurement, care planning was done for nearly 100% of the patients. At the same time, however, the number of patients with a written assessment dropped on three of the four wards from nearly 100% to between 0% and 45%. In these four wards, the reason was seen as insufficient software functionality, which led to slow documentation of an assessment. Subsequently, the nurses failed to produce an assessment; not even returning to the old paper-based forms.

In addition, a significant increase in the number of documented problems, aims and planned interventions was found on all four wards at the third time of measurement, irrespective of whether paper-based care planning had been conducted beforehand or not. For example, the number of documented problems per patient rose from 3.7 to 20.7 on ward A. Similar numbers were found for nursing aims. The number of documented interventions per day also increased significantly on three of the four wards (e.g. from 7.7 to 35.2 on ward C). Interestingly, the numbers during the second measurement point were even higher than those for the last point (e.g. 48.7 daily documented interventions on ward C after 3 months of use). Nurses quickly learnt that this enormous amount of documentation was not feasible and the number then declined after some time. Those results show that nurses need some time to exploit the possibilities of computer-based nursing documentation properly.

The two external reviewers also judged some other aspects of quality (Mahler et al 2005). They often found that problems mentioned in the nursing report could not be found in the care plan. They also found that care plans often were not well adapted to the individual patient ('checklist effect'). This meant that the care plan did not really reflect the situation of the patient, and that it was very often inconsistent with observations given in the assessment or in the reports. Especially in the early stages of IT implementation, nurses seemed not to reflect sufficiently on the given predefined care plans, taking what was given without adapting it to an individual patient. Overall, both reviewers found that the completeness and transparency of the documentation had improved, although they criticized the decrease in individualization in the documentation. Their overall judgment was that the quality of documentation increased only slightly between the first and third measurement points (from 2.8 points to 3.1 points for reviewer A, and from 2.2 to 3.1 points for reviewer B, on a five-point scale).

In conclusion, computer-based nursing documentation can improve many formal aspects of quality, such as readability and completeness. Computer use may also support a more frequent use of the documentation and more frequent updating of care plans. This improvement depends on the quality and flexibility of the computer-based system, on the number and availability of sufficient hardware and, most of all, on the motivation of the users. If these factors are not positive, then IT may lead to less individualized documentation. We will analyse this aspect further in the following section.

IT and the professionalization of nursing care

The introduction of IT may change the way nurses work, but also how they (and others) see their work. In general, nurses often feel that computer skills and computer use are not part of their image of nursing (Adaskin et al 1994). They do, however, often accept computers after the implementation phase as a necessary part of both private and professional life, and may even feel proud of being able to use new technologies. Büssing and Herbig (1998) argued that IT forces nurses to deal with the Nursing Process and related questions, and that computers within nursing education and nursing practice would even improve the general reputation of nursing. This would support professionalization. Computers may also be seen as working against an individualized approach to patient care. Goossen et al (1997) argued that one main problem with nursing information systems is the discrepancy between the care delivery to individuals on the one hand, and the standardization and rationalization of health care owing to IT on the other.

A detailed analysis was carried out by Harris (1990), based on an interview study of 14 nurses who had worked with computerized care planning for several years. He summarized the results in three main parts: First, he found a deprofessionalization of the nurses as a result of using the computer. Nurses felt controlled by the computer, and felt that they were losing skills associated with the 'old' ways of care planning. Second, the nurses felt that care planning was less individualized. While in nursing, individualization of care is highly valued, the software forces nurses to construct care plans from standardized plans, which are often too general really to fit a patient. The possibility of free-text entry, or of selecting or unselecting items, would take more time, and might make the plan too long. Harris (1990) thus argued that free text was often not used by the nurses. Third, he found de-skilling of nurses. They simply used the computer without having to think too much, judging the computerized care planning as fast, easy and convenient, thus losing the documentation skills learned in nursing school. Harris also argued, however, that these de-skilling and deprofessionalization effects are dependent on the environment. They would appear when the nursing care plan (whether computerized or not) was not valued, and when nurses were rewarded more for its existence, than for its quality. He also reported results from another ward, where nurses used a lot of free text, producing highly individualized care plans. Here, the nurses were autonomous and motivated enough to combat the computer's implicit demands for standardized input.

Harris' (1990) results have subsequently been supported by other studies. For example, Larrabee (2001) also found a problem with insufficient individualization of computer-based care plans. Adaskin et al (1994) argued that high-turnover units, such as critical care, often find that patients' needs change too rapidly to allow the entry of changes into computerized care plans. These selected examples accentuate an important point which may be often overlooked when introducing computers in nursing documentation: computers will not miraculously solve all the problems that already exist with paper-based nursing care plans (Newton 1995). Computers can lead to more complete and readable documentation of the Nursing Process, but they may also tempt nurses to be satisfied with this achievement, overlooking the emerging danger of quick, but completely standardized and impersonal care planning, which is overly reliant on care standards already provided.

Harris (1990) concluded that some nurses might consider computer-based documentation to be like 'fast food' – fast, easy and convenient. Nurses must, therefore, be sufficiently trained during the introduction to patient-oriented documentation to use computers to create not only comprehensive but also individualized care plans. Computers can make care plans easier to handle and to update. However, if not correctly applied, they can also lead to documentation weak in individualization. Information technology is only a tool, which can be used or abused. Nursing services should, therefore, first invest in motivation and training of future users, making them willing to invest time in individualized care planning, and then introduce computers to make their life easier and to reduce effort.

IT and user acceptance

The introduction of IT in nursing practice may at first be accompanied by fear and anxiety of the users, but typically, after a time, user acceptance increases as nurses become used to the new technology. For example, Adaskin et al (1994) interviewed ten staff nurse users and ten nurse educators or administrators about 6 months after the introduction of a complete computer-based nursing documentation system, which included the Cardex and an order-entry component. The nurses reported feelings of stress and time pressure, and an increase in workload at the beginning. They worried about risks to patient safety during the chaos and rush of the implementation period. However, after the actual implementation period was over, they tended to view the system more positively.

Many other authors have also reported on high user acceptance of computer-based nursing documentation systems (e.g. Allan and Englebright 2000). Lowry (1994) questioned 54 ICU nurses on their attitudes towards computer-based care planning and found medium to highly positive attitudes. Nurses said that IT was time-saving, and would increase the quality of documentation and individualization of patient care. Getty et al (1999) questioned nurses after 2 years of use of computer-based nursing and found positive statements with regard to more individualization of patient care through computers, an increase in the quality of documentation and a reduction of paperwork.

Pabst et al (1996) reported on focus group interviews on one ward, which implemented a bedside nursing information system. Nurses felt positive about the system, found that their documentation was more complete, readable and accurate, that they could generate care plans more quickly, and that they were able to individualize and update care plans very easily. Negative comments were that there was insufficient integration with the overall electronic patient record system, making nursing progress notes unavailable to other professional groups.

Adaskin et al (1994) found that previous computer experiences clearly affected nurses' feelings about computerization. The higher the personal computer knowledge, the easier it was to learn the new system. This is confirmed by an analysis in Ammenwerth et al (2003) and points to the need for basic computer training in addition to system-specific training prior to the implementation of IT.

On the other hand, strong dissatisfaction is also possible, especially when the system suddenly forces a complete individual care plan, as Newton (1995) argued. Nurses then often complained that computer care planning was inflexible, time consuming, had increased their workload, reduced patient individuality and diminished nurses' autonomy. These complaints often seemed to be related more to care planning in general than to the use of computers. The problems, therefore, seem to occur more often on wards where no paper-based care planning had been done before.

Besides general computer experience, a lot of research has been performed to find other factors, such as age or professional experience, that influence user acceptance of computers. Lowry (1993) found a positive correlation between age, the length of time qualified and the length of time employed on nurses' attitudes towards computerized care plans. Similar studies on influencing factors have been conducted by Marasovic et al (1997), McBride & Nagle (1996), Scarpa et al (1992), Sleutel and Guinn (1999), and Vassar et al (1999). Burkes (1991) questioned 56 nurses on an ICU 1 year after the implementation of a computerized charting program. He could not confirm his hypotheses that age or educational level was correlated to satisfaction with the computerized system. What he found was that nurses who had greater computer experience were less satisfied with computerized charting, which stands in contrast to other papers. This example shows that the combination of various factors that influence user satisfaction is still not sufficiently understood by nursing research. A comprehensive discussion of the often contrasting findings of the literature was provided by Getty et al (1999).

CONCLUSION

Information technology is just a tool, and its effects depend on the way it is used in daily practice. It does not solve all the existing problems with nursing documentation but does offer new possibilities not offered by paper documentation.

The effect of computer-based documentation on the outcome of patient care has not yet been analysed. This correlation will not be easy to prove. The main factor in good patient care is still the competence and motivation of the staff. Computers are just one tool among many to make this job easier or more efficient.

Nursing informatics should be a strong part of nursing education. In the future, nurses increasingly will be confronted with computers in many areas of their professional life. It is important that they are able to understand the basic principles, and to balance both the risks and benefits of computers.

We should not forget that nursing informatics is only one part of clinical informatics. In other words, nursing information and documentation systems can only be one part of an overall electronic patient record. Only the firm integration of several sources of data (from a nursing, physician or other point of view) will lead to a comprehensive patient-related record that comprises all aspects of patient care. This does not mean that we need to neglect the peculiarities of the different professional groups, but we should not, while considering details of nursing informatics, forget the larger picture with the patient at the centre.

REFERENCES

Adaskin E, Hughes L, McMullan P, McLean M, McMorris D 1994 The impact of computerization on nursing: an interview study of users and facilitators. Computers in Nursing 12: 141–149

Allan J, Englebright J 2000 Patient-centered documentation - an effective and efficient use of clinical information systems. Journal of Nursing Administration 30(2): 90–95

Ammenwerth E, Eichstädter R, Haux R, Pohl U, Rebel S, Ziegler S 2001 A randomized evaluation of a computer-based nursing documentation system. Methods of Information in Medicine 40(2): 61–68

Ammenwerth E, Mansmann U, Mahler C, Kandert M, Eichstädter R 2002 Are quantitative methods sufficient to show why wards react differently to computer-based nursing documentation? In: Surjan G et al (eds) Proceedings of the XVIIth International Congress of the European Federation for Medical Informatics (Medical Informatics Europe 2002 – Health Data in the Information Society), 25–29.8.02, Budapest. IOS Press Amsterdam: 377–381

Ammenwerth E, Mansmann U, Iller C, Eichstädter R 2003 Factors affecting and affected by user acceptance of computer-based nursing documentation: results of a two-year study. Journal of the American Medical Informatics Association 10(1): 69–84

Burkes M 1991 Identifying and relating nurses' attitudes toward computer use. Computers in Nursing 9(5): 190–201

Bürkle T, Kuch R, Prokosch H, Dudeck J 1999 Stepwise evaluation of information systems in a university hospital. Method of Information in Medicine 38(1): 9–15

Büssing A, Herbig B 1998 The challenges of a care information systems reflecting holistic nursing care. Computers in Nursing 16(6): 311–317

Davis B, Billings J, Ryland R 1994 Evaluation of nursing process documentation. Journal of Advanced Nursing 19(5): 960–968

Getty M, Ryan A, Ekins M 1999 A comparative study of the attitudes of users and non-users towards computerized care planning. Journal of Clinical Nursing 8: 431–439

Goossen W, Epping P, Dassen T, Hasman A, van den Heuvel W 1997 Can we solve current problems with nursing information systems? Computer Methods Programs Biomedicine 54(1, 2): 85–91

Hannah K J, Ball M J, Edwards M J 1999 Introduction to nursing informatics. Springer, New York

Harris B 1990 Becoming de-professionalized: One aspect of the staff nurse's perspective on computer-mediated nursing care plans. Advances in Nursing Science 13(2): 63–74

Kahl K, Ivancin L, Fuhrmann M 1991 Automated nursing documentation system provides a favorable return on investment. Journal of Nursing Administration 21(11): 44–51

Larrabee J 2001 Evaluation of documentation before and after implementation of a nursing information system in an acute care hospital. Computers in Nursing 19(2): 56–65

Leiner F, Haux R 1996 Systematic planning of clinical documentation: Methods of Information Medicine 35: 25–34

Lichten E, Soble I 1984 A microcomputer nursing workstation. Journal of Clinical Engineering 9(2): 135–140

Lowry C 1994 Nurses' attitudes toward computerised care plans in intensive care. Part 2. Intensive and Critical Care Nursing 10: 2–11

Lowry H 1993 Nurses' attitudes toward computerised care plans in intensive care. Part 1. Intensive and Critical Care Nursing 9: 242–245

Mahler C, Ammenwerth E, Eichstädter R et al 2002 Evaluation eines rechnergestützten Pflegedokumentationssystems. Evaluation of a Computer-based nursing documentation system – final report. Research report: University Hospitals of Heidelberg, Germany

Mahler C, Ammenwerth E, Wagner A et al 2005 Effects of a computer-based nursing documentation system on the quality of nursing documentation. Journal of Medical Systems (accepted for publication)

Marasovic C, Kenney C, Elliott D, Sindhusake D 1997 Attitudes of Australian nurses toward the implementation of a clinical information system. Computers in Nursing 15(2): 91–98

McBride S, Nagle L 1996 Attitudes towards computers: A test of construct validity. Computers in Nursing 14: 164–170

Newton C 1995 A study of nurses' attitudes and quality of documents in computer care planning. Nursing Standard 9: 35–39

Pabst M K, Scherubel J C, Minnick A F 1996 The impact of computerized documentation on nurses' use of time. Computers Nursing 14(1): 25–30

Pryor T A 1989 Computerized nurse charting. International Journal on Clinical Monitoring and Computing 6(3): 173–179

Romano C, McCormick K, McNeely L 1982 Nursing documentation: a model for a computerized data base. Advances in Nursing Science 2: 43–56

Saba V K 1997 A look at nursing informatics: International Journal of Medical Information 44(1): 57–60

Scarpa R, Smeltzer S, Jasion B 1992 Attitudes of nurses toward computerization. A replication. Computers in Nursing 10(2): 72–80

Sleutel M, Guinn M, 1999 As good as it gets? Going online with a clinical information system. Computers in Nursing 17(4): 181–185

van Gennip E, Klaassen-Leil C, Stokman R, van Valkenburg R 1995 Costs and effects of a nursing information system in three Dutch hospitals. In: Greenes R et al (eds) Medinfo 95 – Proceedings of the 8th World Congress on Medical Informatics. North Holland, Amsterdam: 1412–1416

Vassar J A, Binshan L, Planckock N 1999 Nursing information systems: a survey of current practices. Top Health Information Management 19(4): 58–65

Chapter 6

The Nursing Process: core of nursing? A Finnish perspective

Maritta Välimäki and Marja Kaunonen

INTRODUCTION

In this paper, we discuss the development and meaning of the Nursing Process in Finland. First, a background to the development of vocational and academic education in Finland will be presented. Second, we offer some landmarks for the establishment of nursing research that have provided new opportunities for nurses to use the Nursing Process in everyday practice. Third, different definitions of the concept of the Nursing Process used in research studies and textbooks will be given. Fourth, implementation of the use of the Nursing Process in everyday clinical practice and its impact on current nursing will be described, together with the problems that nurses have faced. Lastly, future challenges for nursing will be discussed. In doing this, we hope to offer an overview of how the Nursing Process has been interpreted and implemented in Finland.

BACKGROUND TO VOCATIONAL AND ACADEMIC NURSING EDUCATION IN FINLAND

In Finland, nursing education began in 1867 when the Helsinki Deaconess Institute was founded. The model for education was taken from the German Kaiserswerth. In accordance with the German model, Finland's first deaconess institute treated the sick and trained deaconesses, helped the poor and took care of homeless children (Helsinki Deaconess Institute 2003). According to other sources, nursing education was started in Finland in 1889 with courses at the Helsinki General Hospital (Helsingin yleinen sairaala) to educate nurses for the whole of Finland.

Early Finnish nursing leaders, Anna Broms, Sophie Mannerheim and Ellen Nylander, received an important part of their education with close connections to Florence Nightingale. Anna Broms studied in Edinburgh Royal Infirmary but she visited St Thomas Hospital. She later worked as the first director of nursing at the Helsinki New Surgical Hospital. Sophie Mannerheim studied in the Nightingale school from 1899 to 1902 and worked as the Director of Nursing in the Helsinki Surgical Hospital. In the Finnish perspective, Sophie Mannerheim can be seen as the Finnish equivalent to Florence Nightingale. The London Hospital was Ellen Nylander's place of study prior to her work as the first matron of the preparatory nursing school (Sorvettula 1998). This early international collaboration may have had an impact on the application of the Nursing Process in nurses' thinking and education in Finland.

In 1910, the Nursing Staff Act (AK 25/1910) formed the basis for the registration of nurses. In 1915, The National Board of Health began the registration of educated nurses. The first Act (AK 340/1929) and bylaw statute (AK 424/1929) came into force in 1929 to regulate nursing education. It was introduced internationally in International Nursing Review in 1930. Formerly, nurses and their responsibilities were regulated by byelaw statutes.

The Finnish Association of Nurses was founded in 1925. Before that, Swedish-speaking nurses had their own organization, Sjuksköterske-föreningen i Finland (Finnish Nursing Association), which was founded in

1898. Finnish nurses were actively following international trends but it was only in 1909 that their organization became a member of the International Council for Nurses (ICN), although Sophie Mannerheim had already been named as Honorary Vice-President in 1907. An ICN meeting was later organized in Helsinki in 1925 (Sorvettula 1998). Finnish nurses were influenced by international experiences of nursing care. In 1938, Florence Nightingale's *Notes on nursing* was translated into Finnish (Nightingale, 1987). Later, the first trade unions for nurses and public health nurses, together with the Education Foundation of Nurses, were founded in 1944 (Lauri 1990a).

New legislation for nursing education was developed at the end of the 1960s, when nursing education was transferred under the National Board of Vocational Education. The reformed regulations were concerned with nursing registration and education and also governed other professionals as well (Health Care Professionals Act 554/1962). In general, the 1960s was a time for development of the Finnish education system and public well-being. This allowed nursing education at university level to begin to develop (Sinkkonen 1999).

During the late 1950s and 1960s, there was much public debate in Finland about academic nursing education and nursing research (Sinkkonen 1988, Lauri 1990a). Landmarks in the history of nursing research include the publishing of the *Yearbook of nursing* in 1958. The Research Institute of Nursing was founded in 1966 (Leino-Kilpi and Suominen 1998). The mission of the institute was to conduct scientific research in nursing and health care and to provide training for researchers in the field (Lauri 1990a).

The 1970s can be described as a very active decade in terms of debate and basic research in nursing science (Leino-Kilpi and Suominen 1998). In the early 1970s, nurses were consciously encouraged to study in Finland in disciplines closely related to nursing, rather than travel abroad for study (Lauri 1990a). In 1979, the University of Kuopio was the first university in Finland to start a degree programme in health administration with nursing science as a major (Sinkkonen 1988). This has made it possible for registered nurses to enhance their knowledge base in the field of nursing science.

During the 1980s, the analysis of concepts and thinking in the field of nursing science became more systematic (Leino-Kilpi and Suominen 1998). By this time, the discipline of nursing science had also become fairly well established (Kalkas 1982). The early 1980s was the period of the establishment of academic education for nurses in Finland. Following the University of Kuopio, nursing science has been taught at university level at the University of Tampere since 1981, originally under the Faculty of Medicine and, from 1990, in the Department of Nursing Science (University of Tampere 2003). The University of Turku's Department of Nursing Science was founded in 1986 as a part of the Faculty of Medicine (University of Turku 2003). Also, at Oulu University, education at the Department of Nursing and Health Administration began in 1986 (University of Oulu 2003). The goal was to educate registered nurses, and to offer them an opportunity for scientific thinking and increase their opportunities for performing research in nursing.

THE DEVELOPMENT OF THE NURSING PROCESS IN FINLAND

Even before the concept of the Nursing Process was officially launched in Finland in the 1970s, the concept 'hoitotapahtuma' (nursing action) was used to describe the actions and processes in social and health care. For example, in 1967, the most central nursing textbook *Sairaanhoito-oppi* (Vetelä-suo 1967) described nursing action, which included four phases: patient analysis, prioritization of the different domains of nursing, selection of the care mode and nursing care. Eriksson (1977: 9–10) defined nursing action as an intervention process, which included patient analysis, definition of the nursing domains, selection of the care modes, nursing care and process factors.

However, process thinking was not introduced into health care from the discipline of nursing. In the 1970s, the National Board of Health (Suomen Lääkintöhallitus) gave written guidelines for patient medical records in both general (Sairaalaliitto 1980) and psychiatric hospitals (Sairaalaliitto 1979). Medical doctors had a responsibility to keep written medical records including descriptions of a patient's state of illness, exploration and treatment plan, as well as implemented examinations and treatments. Other staff had their own pages in the records.

The concept of the Nursing Process can be found in Finnish nursing debates in the 1960s (e.g. Leminen 1966). At that time, there were rapid changes in Finnish society and health care organizations owing to the development of medicine and medical technology. New groups of professions were introduced into health care and tasks were moved from one profession to another. After these changes, nurses started to ask themselves what their role was in health care. The application of process thinking to nursing was perceived as providing answers to those questions (Savolainen and Kärki 1983).

The first research worker and director of the Research Institute (Aili Leminen) studied the topic 'What do nurses do?' Between 1968 and 1972, she presented papers mainly discussing topics related to nurses' work. Lauri (1990a) stated that Leminen's paper 'On the Nursing Process and its research', which was published in 1973, raised a lot of new ideas in Finland and was also published in Swedish. The paper was also seen as an official starting point of the Nursing Process in Finland. In 1975, a research project called the 'Development of models and methods of the Nursing Process' was started by Professor Hertta Kalkas, with Sirkka Lauri as a researcher.

However, it has been stated that, instead of perceiving process thinking as a model describing nursing action, it was seen first as a normative guideline for action. It was thought to indicate what nursing should be and how it should be implemented (Sinkkonen and Savolainen 1983). Later, the application of process thinking in nursing led to the development of several process models as well as their implementation in the Nursing Process. For example, Eriksson (1989) turns Nursing Process thinking upside down or backwards. She discussed the Nursing Process in her writings from the viewpoint of health and defined the Nursing Process as a means to achieve health: health is the goal of the Nursing Process. Her focus is strongly on a person not on a nurse's action. Parviainen (1992: 100), instead of the Nursing Process, discusses 'logical continuation in health and nursing care', although using the familiar concepts from the Nursing Process – need definition, planning, nursing action and nursing evaluation.

However, in different models of the Nursing Process, the background is the same, that is, with different phases or steps to organize systematic nursing (Savolainen and Kärki 1984). For example, Lauri introduced a rational–analytical model in her research about decision-making in nursing (e.g. Lauri 1982a, 1982b, 1984, 1985). Five phases included in her nursing and health care process can be seen in her early work: information collection, problem definition, planning of actions, implementation of action and evaluation (Lauri 1977, 1991, see Lauri et al 1998). Professor Lauri also has an important role in the project implemented in North Karelia Central Hospital, where the concept of decision-making was named as the Nursing Process (Lauri 1982a). The concept of the Nursing Process used in this project was derived particularly from the World Health Organisation (WHO; 1977) definition. She also introduced the idea of the Nursing Process in her later research (Lauri 1982b).

Different studies provided knowledge concerning the Nursing Process for nursing students and nursing practice. Together with nursing textbooks, there was a lot of information about the concept of the Nursing Process and how it has been defined in Finland. In 1979, Kalkas and colleagues published a definition of the Nursing Process as a system characteristic of nursing consisting of actions towards an individual's, a family's and/or a community's health. It includes identification of a patient's/client's/family's/community's health needs using scientific methods, selection of the needs most effective assessed with nursing action, as well as planning how to meet the needs, the nursing care and evaluating the results of the process (Kalkas et al 1979, Savolainen and Kärki 1983).

Heiskanen and Huopalahti (1984) described the Nursing Process as an instrument with which clinical nursing care is analysed and implemented. It is a problem-solving process that helps nurses with their decision-making (Hentinen 1984). It includes a definition of nursing care needs, planning the care, implementing the care and evaluating it. Lauri (1991) defined the Nursing Process as conscious and active thinking and decision-making, based on the needs of the patients. Iivanainen et al (1995) have also seen the Nursing Process as an instrument for analytical thinking which supports planning of nursing care, and implementing and evaluating it. It is an interaction based on problem-solving and decision making aimed towards identifying and reaching the nursing goals.

Several English-language textbooks related to the Nursing Process were used for nursing education in Finland. Some examples are LaMonica's (1979) *The Nursing Process: a humanistic approach* and Marriner's (1979) *The Nursing Process: a scientific approach to nursing care*. Other nursing textbooks, translated from their original language (mainly English), were also used (e.g. Kratz 1993). The fourth edition of *The Nursing Process: assessing, planning, implementing, evaluating* by Yura and Walsh was translated into Finnish in 1988. In the foreword, it is acknowledged that, when the first edition was published in 1967 and the second in 1973, they were the only publications using the concept of the Nursing Process. However, by the time the Finnish version was published, the Nursing Process was a topic covered in nearly all nursing textbooks. The Research Institute of Nursing is the publisher of the book and, in the foreword to the Finnish edition, they hope the book will advance the dynamic development of nursing in Finland. It was also noted that nursing knowledge had increased over the years and, therefore, readers needed to use critical thinking when reading the book. The Finnish version of the book gained wide popularity and, for several years, was one of the books used for admission tests for departments of nursing science at different Finnish universities.

HOW THE NURSING PROCESS HAS BEEN IMPLEMENTED IN NURSING RESEARCH AND EVERYDAY NURSING PRACTICE

In the 1970s and 1980s, the Nursing Process became a natural part of the curriculum of colleges of nursing. Nursing students practised the use of care plans for patients using the Nursing Process as the framework for care applied to individual patients. The Nursing Process was also used as a framework of care in seminar papers and assignments.

The Nursing Process was acknowledged and used by academics in their studies and publications. Krause provided an assessment of the quality of nursing and presented her thoughts diagrammatically (Figure 6.1). These were originally published in Finnish (Krause 1983) and later in English (Krause and Kiikkala 1992). Krause (1984) noticed that the use of the Nursing Process can be seen to systematize nursing care, but she questioned whether its implementation could lead to individuality in patient care (Krause 1984, Tuomi 1997). The Nursing Process model was implemented in doctoral dissertations as well. The first doctoral dissertation in nursing science in Finland was Hentinen's development project at the Kuopio University Hospital between 1980 and 1982 ('Developing a programme of nursing care for patients with myocardiac infarction at Kuopio University Hospital, 1980–1982'). Hentinen's (1984) central perspective to nursing has been that of the Nursing Process. She reminds us that the Nursing Process as a process method only provides the logical structure for nursing and does not provide, for example, nursing principles along which to act.

By the end of the 1980s, nursing science attempted to establish its place among other disciplines and altogether four individuals have completed doctoral dissertations in health care with majors in nursing science. Besides Hentinen's dissertation, the other three are 'The entirety of a population's health care: self-care, utilization of official and unofficial health care services and their determinants in Finland' (1986) by Meriläinen; 'Getting cancer: adapting to the changing life situation' (1987) by Krause; and 'Supervision in nursing' (1989) by Paunonen (Lauri 1990a).

One indication of the level of academic nursing was the foundation of the Association of Caring Sciences (Hoitotieteiden tutkimusseura ry; HTTS) in Kuopio in 1987. The purpose of this association is to support and promote research in nursing science and its applications in clinical nursing. It also organizes national and international scientific conferences, and administers grants for research and publishing. The association publishes a scientific

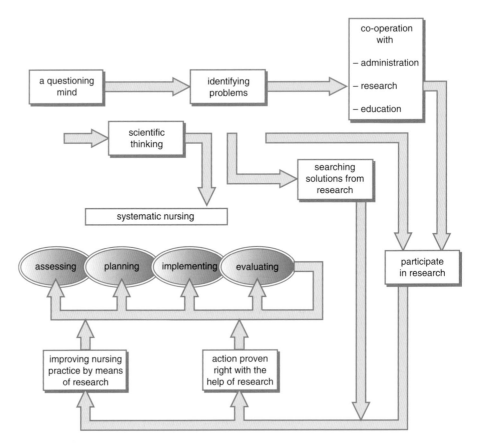

Figure 6.1 Nurses and their research-based practice (Source: Krause 1983, Krause and Kiikkala 1992: 30)

journal in Finnish, *Hoitotiede* (*Journal of Nursing Science*), which was established in 1989, and promotes regional activity (HTTS 2003).

In the 1990s, a doctoral dissertation by Kaija Nojonen (1990) entitled 'The rehabilitation of a long-term patient' was implemented in the North Häme mental health care district. It was part of the Finnish National Programme for the Treatment and Rehabilitation of Schizophrenic Patients and was initiated in 1985. The structure used in the rehabilitation plans of the long-term psychiatric patients was the Nursing Process model. This multiprofessional, national-level study indicates that the Nursing Process was accepted and applied as the basis of nursing care not only by nurses but also other professionals.

How was the Nursing Process implemented in everyday nursing practice? Unfortunately, studies conducted between the 1970s and 1990s do not directly support the statement that different phases of the Nursing Process had been included in nurses' work. A study conducted in 1976 showed that 65–69 % of public health nurses estimated that their collection of information physical needs and health problems of children was well implemented (Lauri 1977). Altogether 53% described that they do planning of action and implementation well, but only 20% evaluated their nursing care. In general, the decision-making process of public health nurses was based on children's physical needs. The results were very similar when the study was repeated ten years later (Lauri 1982a, 1986, Hyvönen and Lauri 1988, Liuksila 1991).

Later studies related to nurses' roles and written care plan documents showed that the goals for nursing are not defined, and the efficacy of nursing interventions is not evaluated or is done only on a small scale (Nissinen 1978, Hentinen et al 1979). For example, public health nurses working with children are knowledgeable about different phases in the Nursing Process. However, the goal of nursing care and evaluations are lacking (Lauri 1990b). Other studies have also shown that the phases of the Nursing Process are known but were not obvious in written nursing documentation (Liuksila 1991, Lehti 2000). Nurses working with psychogeriatric patients evaluated that identification of nursing problems was carried out properly, but over half the nurses indicated that evaluation of patients' nursing is done only moderately or poorly. Analysis of the content of care plans revealed the inadequacy of the written plans (Liukkonen 1989).

A project at one university hospital indicated that the written documentation of nursing was done poorly in spite of the fact that written documentation had been the topic of training/education for several years in the hospital. Nursing problems were identified quite well but the goals of nursing care were documented poorly. Implementation of nursing in comparison with the patient's problems and the effectiveness of nursing could not be identified in 30% of the patient documents. In comparison, evaluation of the nursing goals and results could be done on only 21% of the documents. An outsider evaluating the documents was able to obtain some kind of holistic view from the Nursing Process in altogether 30% of written patient documents (Lauri 1991).

DEVELOPING THE QUALITY AND THE QUANTITY OF NURSING EDUCATION AND RESEARCH AT THE TURN OF THE CENTURY

The 1990s was the decade of rapid change in the Finnish health care system. Finland was economically in depression, which had an enormous effect on health care and nursing. At the same time, nursing education changed dramatically. In 1992, a programme of polytechnic education in nursing was piloted and, by the end of 1998, the education of registered nurses was totally transformed under the polytechnics. An attempt was made to increase the collaboration between nursing practice and education. The basic idea was that research experience obtained during nursing education increases nurses' opportunities for research-based practice and practitioner-based research (Hankela 1999).

In the 1990s, nursing science gained a solid position in Finland. In 1996, seven university-level master and doctoral programmes were offered at the Universities of Helsinki, Tampere, Kuopio, Oulu, Turku, Jyväskylä and Åbo Akademin (Vaasa). By the beginning of September 1999, almost 2000 masters, 153 licentiates and 86 doctors in nursing science had graduated in Finland (Sinkkonen 1999). Universities had different research branches:

family nursing and mental health nursing in University of Tampere; acute clinical or geriatric clinical, or clinical nursing and elderly care in Turku; nursing administration, radiography and laboratory science in Oulu; preventive nursing science research and education in Kuopio; and caring science, health care administration and the didactics of care in Åbo Akademin in Vaasa, mainly in the Swedish language.

In general, the primary focus of nursing research in the 1990s was clinical and reflects the broad range of issues that have been covered in the short history of nursing research in Finland. Closely related to clinical research was work developing different models of action, such as Nursing Process methods and the transformation of nursing practices from being task-oriented to patient-oriented (Suominen and Leino-Kilpi 1998). The Nursing Process was no longer used as much in nursing, and criticism towards it existed. It was said to stress the role of the nurse in the decision-making and to emphasize the role of the patient too little (Krause and Salo 1992). It was also thought to lead nursing to become routinized and ritualized (e.g. Kiikkala 1998). In doctoral dissertations (e.g. Leino-Kilpi 1990, Liukkonen 1990, Ollikainen 1994, Välimäki 1998) and other publications, qualitative methods were used to gain a deeper understanding of everyday reality in nursing.

On the other hand, the idea of the Nursing Process has still been used in different research contexts (e.g. as a part of action research). In Munnukka's doctoral dissertation (1993) 'From functional nursing to primary nursing', the elements of the action research process and the Nursing Process can be found as a process of thinking and problem-solving. The researcher stated that her results point to differences between functional nursing and primary nursing in how the Nursing Process was realized. It was noteworthy that most of the patients interviewed in the study indicated that they were not involved in the care planning, when the aims of their care were discussed or even when the decisions concerning their care were made.

In mental health nursing, Latvala and Janhonen (1996) published their article 'Patient's management in daily life – basic process of psychiatric nursing in hospital environment'. Their results indicated that the basis of psychiatric nursing was to care for the needs of the patient, in which different methods of nursing were utilized. The study report lacks the description of evaluation of the Nursing Process, although the researchers highlight the need for further study in the area of nurses' perception of evaluation (Latvala and Janhonen 1996).

In his doctoral thesis, Jouni Tuomi (1997) has analysed and described the Finnish debate in nursing and caring science from before the 1970s to the beginning of the 1990s (1968–1991). The arguments in nursing and caring science were based on reviews of the literature from seven experts on nursing and caring science who held posts as professors in Finland during 1991. The experts were: Hertta Kalkas; Sirkka Sinkkonen; Emerita Professors of Nursing Sciences Sirkka Lauri, Maija Hentinen, Marita Paunonen (later Paunonen-Ilmonen) Kaisa Krause and Katie Eriksson. The analysis showed that the basis for the development of the discussion and use of the 'Nursing Process' concept was the WHO definition of the Nursing Process from the year 1977 and the rational–analytical model of action. The use of

WHO concepts and the rational–analytical model of thinking was later shifted to a wider perspective in Lauri's research, when she introduced decision-making theory from the phenomenological viewpoint in 1991 (Tuomi 1997).

WHERE ARE WE TODAY?

Today, the Finnish higher education system consists of two sectors: universities and polytechnics. The polytechnics are more practically oriented, training professionals for expert and development posts. There are 29 polytechnics in Finland; most are multidisciplinary, regional institutions, which give particular weight to contacts with business and industry. The Ministry of Education confirms professional qualifications, degrees, the degree programmes and the number of new students. The polytechnics award professionally oriented higher education degrees, which take 3.5 or 4 years. The entry requirement is either an upper secondary school certificate or a vocational diploma. At present, about 70% of all entrants are matriculated students and 30% vocational graduates. There is no tuition fee for degree studies (Ministry of Education 2003). Polytechnics are developed as part of the national and international higher education community, with special emphasis on their expertise in working life and its development. The polytechnics also carry out R&D relevant to their teaching and to the world of work.

At 31 December 2002, a total of 59 322 registered nurses lived in Finland. In addition, 2334 nurses had a further degree: 598 in health care administration and 1736 in education (nursing teacher) (Terveydenhuollon oikeusturvakeskus 2002). University-level master's degrees (in general, a compulsory prerequisite to a nurse's training) are offered at the universities of Tampere, Kuopio, Oulu, Turku and Åbo Akademi (Vaasa). At the present time, master's studies in administration-oriented health care with nursing science as the major subject can also be taken in Tampere, Kuopio and Oulu. University education leads to the qualification of Master of Nursing Science (MNSc), which is a higher academic degree. It consists of 240 European Credit Transfer System (ECTS) credits (or 160 credits in the Finnish University system). Previous vocational education is acceptable as a substitute for a proportion of the coursework. The departments also offer postgraduate programmes leading to licentiate's or doctor's degree. There is also a national doctoral programme in nursing, which is run jointly by all universities.

The idea of the Nursing Process can also be seen in modern health technology. For example, the content and structure of patient electronic records are often based on the Nursing Process (Iivanainen et al 1995). Electronic patient records are expected to produce better quality documentation, improve patients' total care in different phases of the care (Saranto 1998a), and make it possible to save patients' nursing plans in their personal electronic records or their e-Health cards (Lauharanta and Rotonen 1998). However, Lehtikunnas and colleagues (2002) indicated that studies on computed-based documentation have shown that computer-based systems lack the support of documentation from the Nursing Process. Their study results also revealed that there was not even one patient's care plan finished when patient documents were analysed after 24 hours. On the other hand, nursing aims or problems were identified in almost half of the cases, which again support studies carried out almost 30 years earlier. They concluded that nurses documented the implementation of medical care well but that nursing care received less attention.

An electronic patient record file can offer online information on the health status of the patient and allow the information to be used in decision-making for nursing diagnoses, interventions and outcomes (Saranto 1998a). Giving a nursing diagnosis to a patient has not gained popularity thus far in Finland, neither has choosing the patient's nursing diagnosis from a readymade list been recognized as a task for his or her nurse. However, the use of the nursing diagnosis process as well as education about its use will become more important in future in Finland (Hallila 1998). There are good grounds for this: Saranto (1998b) in her study reports that student nurses showed a positive attitude towards computer use in health care. Today, electronic patient records are used in a number of health care centres in Finland and are in the development process in all five university hospitals.

One indication of the status of nursing science in Finland is the semi-annual national nursing science conference that is organized in collaboration with one department of nursing science at a time and the Finnish Association of Caring Sciences (Hoitotieteiden tutkimusseura ry). The participants represent a large number of Finnish academic nurses, as well as those working in clinical settings, and the presentations each year provide a good view of Finnish nursing research. For this report, the proceedings book of the national conference in Oulu in October 2002 was analysed by means of the Nursing Process. The proceedings book contained 44 articles in all. Analysis revealed that the Nursing Process was either mentioned directly or could be identified in only six papers.

Gardner and colleagues (2002) studied the discharge process for an elderly patient. In their article, the process was derived into four phases: (1) evaluation of the discharge process; (2) discharge decision; (3) organization of the discharge; and (4) evaluation of the success of the discharge process. They also noted that the nurse collaborating in the discharge process worked in a four-phase process. Firstly, the nurse evaluated the life situation of the elderly patient and, secondly, the nurse collaborated with the elderly patient, significant others and other professionals, jointly making a decision concerning the placement of the elderly patient following hospitalization. Thirdly, the discharge was implemented and the fourth phase included the nurse's evaluation of the discharge process. Another study, by Kiikkala and colleagues (2002), considered patient centredness, which was implemented as an action research where all its phases could be identified. Lehtikunnas and colleagues (2002) discussed computer-based documentation and how it fails to support the Nursing Process. The study by Niskanen et al (2002) formed part of the European Early Promotion Project, in which interaction with families and public health nurses in maternal care clinics started with discussion during which possible problems were identified. This paper does not indicate how the interaction continues or whether a process model was used. The Nursing Process was also included in the study questions of Pellikka et al (2002): 'From the patients' view how is the Nursing Process implemented in emergency room?' and 'What is the relationship between the background variables and the implication of the Nursing Process?' Also, in the study results of Sarajärvi and Isola (2002), the work of a nursing student working independently was described with the help of the Nursing Process. The analysis of these studies revealed that the Nursing Process was currently in use, albeit infrequently, but as a basis of nursing work in several different contexts.

The most recent reference to the implementation of Nursing Process in research and clinical practice can be found in the abstract book of the International Conference of Mental Health, which was held in May 2003 in Tampere. The Nursing Process appeared in the presentation 'Syöpäpotilaan osallistuminen päätöksentekoon' by Sainio (2003). The presentation described the participation of a cancer patient of working age in the decision-making process and considered the variables that affected this decision-making. The Nursing Process was also mentioned in a discussion about rehabilitation, in which process thinking was seen as a framework (Hannikainen and Leppänen 2003).

The main characteristics of the Nursing Process can be recognized in the study by Perälä et al (2003). The theme was 'Aim for a client's good hospital discharge and home care'. In the development work, the researchers acknowledged that they implemented care/case management ideology by setting out their work in steps: (1) a client's care path was described; (2) shortcomings in the care path were acknowledged and new solutions were sought; (3) new solutions were described and tested; and (4) new solutions were evaluated in practice. The similarity to the Nursing Process is evident, even though the terms and concepts used differ.

Different phases that include elements of the Nursing Process are seen in different studies in Finland. Process thinking is applied as a framework in several different modes in nursing as a problem-solving circle: collecting information, planning and defining relevant objectives, implementing actual interventions, and evaluating the results (e.g. Pitkänen et al 2003). The focus of the project is to upgrade the managerial skills of the deputy ward sisters in a psychiatric hospital.

In the 2000s, the main focus was on evaluating the effectiveness of care. Several researchers in Finland have also acknowledged the need for practical tools for the health care service and nursing care in its dynamic state, involving both great organizational changes and radical economic cutbacks, to ensure the effectiveness and the quality of care (Mattila et al 2000). Systems of patient classification have been developed as a method for measuring patients' need for help and effective staff planning capable of responding to patients' constantly changing need for care (e.g. Fagerstöm and Rainio 1999, Karhe 2003). As a precondition for nurses to carry out classification of patients, Karhe (2003) stated that nurses' motivation and knowledge of patients increase their recognition of the patients' individual need for help, and also allows that need to be fulfilled. It is remarkable to find that today's problem definitions are produced by collaboration between the patient and the nurse, possibly with the help of the patient's family members. She also recognized the independent decision-making of a primary nurse in an intensive care unit as well as the coordinating role of the primary nurse.

Another challenge for the future is evidence-based nursing (Lauri 2003). As in medicine, the need for different recommendations or guiding principles has also been acknowledged in nursing. In order to implement and apply research knowledge in clinical nursing practice, the Finnish Nurses Association has founded an expert group, which has the task of supporting the development of nursing recommendations for care in Finland. In addition, in 2003, a new nursing journal, *Tutkiva Hoitotyö*, was founded with the aim to help the application of nursing research in practice.

Multinational collaboration, both in the area of developing nursing education and research, has also increased. Most recently, this has been achieved by the 'Tuning Phase II' programme, which aims to understand nursing curricula in different European countries and to make them comparable. The Tuning project has its roots in the Bologna Declaration. The project aims to facilitate the mobility of professionals and degree holders in Europe by finding common points of reference and focusing on competency and skills based on knowledge that professionals have obtained after completing their education (Gonzáles and Wagner 2003). The Department of Nursing Science at the University of Tampere has been involved in this interesting collaboration.

DISCUSSION AND CONCLUSIONS

Process thinking in nursing and the Nursing Process was introduced in Finnish nursing soon after it was developed in the nursing world. Over the decades, several generations of nursing students have studied nursing and patient care with the help of the Nursing Process. The early establishment of academic research and education has provided the basis for the use of scientific thinking by nurses in Finland. In addition, the Nursing Process has served as a framework for scientific research, mainly from the 1970s to the 1990s, and process thinking can still be found in the background of several studies. This development may provide a knowledge base that encourages nurses to use the Nursing Process in their practice and research.

During their nursing education and practice, nurses have learned the Nursing Process as a basis of patient care. Nurses who have studied the Nursing Process in their nursing education or as on-the-job training are now practising nursing. Research results over the last 30 years have shown that different phases including the Nursing Process have been identified in nursing practice. We are still unsure why these phases are not apparent in the nursing documentation; nursing evaluation, particularly, has not been noticed. Also more and more public criticism has been directed towards the Nursing Process, and its drawbacks were already obvious at the beginning of the 1980s (e.g. Sinkkonen and Savolainen 1983).

Because of the economic situation, the evaluation of health care is currently under scrutiny and nurses are required to master different methods related to the effectiveness of care. This means that future challenges are evident in nursing. First, in nursing education, defining the qualification requirements for the nursing profession must be taken into account, requirements based on the regulation of practising health care professions, as well as coordinating the general and specialized skills needed in health care. Besides the core skills, attention must be paid to the future needs for qualifications based on research, health needs of the population and health policy lines, as well as practical training. The qualification requirements for public health nurses and midwives must be defined so that they are based on nursing education and the option chosen within it that is suitable for work as a public health nurse or midwife. Defining the qualification requirements requires close cooperation between education and working life. Second, future requirements for nursing knowledge and challenges for education involve multiprofessional working skills, health promotion, patients, family and community-centred nursing, development of expertise and evidence-based methods. Entrepreneurship in social and health care, application of information technology and telematics, and international collaboration and mobility of nurses within the European Union area as well as globally are important areas for the future. Thus, future challenges in nursing practice are focused on global questions. However, we still believe that systematic thinking has an important role in nursing practice and discipline to ensure the provision of high-quality nursing care.

We can conclude that, as with any other phenomenon, the Nursing Process is a product of its time. Its development, implementation and application as well as its real advantage for nursing and for supporting the wellbeing of people may be a sum of many factors. The main advantage of using the Nursing Process has been that nursing students and nurses have worked systematically in collaboration with the patients and their families, collecting data, defining the nursing needs, implementing nursing and, although less often, evaluating the implemented care. On the other hand, nurses in Finland have also learned to see the drawbacks to the Nursing Process and even express their opinions critically.

REFERENCES

Eriksson K 1977 Hoitotapahtuma. Sairaanhoitajien koulutussäätiö, Helsinki

Eriksson K 1989 Terveyden idea. Sairaanhoitajien koulutussäätiö, Helsinki

Fagerström L, Rainio A-K 1999 Professional assessment of optimal nursing care intensity level: a new method of assessing personnel resources for nursing care. Journal of Clinical Nursing 8: 369–379

Gardner S, Kiviniemi K, Arve S 2002 Vanhuksen kotiutusprosessin elementit – kuvaus kotiutushoitajan toiminnasta. In: Kanste O, Kyngäs H, Lukkarinen H, Utriainen K (eds) Yksilöiden terveyden ja hyvinvoinnin vahvistaminen eri ympäristöissä elämänkulun kaikissa vaiheissa. VII kansallinen hoitotieteellinen konferenssi, Oulu: 24–28

Gonzáles J, Wagner R (eds) 2003 Tuning educational structures in Europe. Final report, Phase One, Universidad de Deusto

Hallila L 1998 Hoitotyön kirjallinen suunnitelma. Kirjayhtymä Oy, Helsinki

Hankela S 1999 Intraoperatiivinen hoitotyö. Empiiriseen aineistoon perustuvan teorian kehittäminen. [Intraoperative nursing development of nursing theory based on empirical data.] (English abstract.) Academic dissertation. Acta Universitatis Tamperensis, Vol. 664, University of Tampere, Finland

Hannikainen T, Leppänen L 2003 Hoitotyön ammattikieli osana moniammatillista viestintää. In: Montin L (ed.) Sairaanhoitajapäivät 2003 Luentotiivistelmät (Finnish Nursing Congress and Exhibition 03, Abstract book), Helsinki

Heiskanen E, Huopalahti P 1984 Hoitotyön avainkäsitteitä. In: Sairaanhoitajien koulutussäätiö. Hoito-opin perusteet. Vaasa Oy, Vaasa, 74–88

Helsinki Deaconess Institute 2003 Available: http://www.hdl.fi/english/history/index.html 25 June 2003

Hentinen M 1984 Sydäninfarktipotilaan hoitotyön kehittämisohjelma Kuopioin yliopistollisen keskussairaalan sisätautien klinikalla 1980–1982. Kuopioin yliopiston iulkaisuja. Yhteiskuntatieteet. Alkuperäistutkimukset 1/1984, Kuopio

Hentinen M, Eronen M, Kiiski M, Nurminen T, Saira H 1979 Hoitotön kirjaaminen: hoitosuunnitelma – ja seurantalomakkeiden arviointi. Sairaanhoidon Vuosikirja XVI. Sairaanhoitajien koulutussäätiö, Helsinki

HTTS [Finnish Association of Caring Sciences] 2003 Available: http://www.uku.fi/htts/englanti.html 8 July 2003

Hyvönen K, Lauri S 1988 Terveydenhoitajan työ ja päätöksentekoprosessi lastenneuvolassa. Toiminnan kehittäminen vuosina 1976–1986. Lääkintöhallituksen julkaisuja 115, Helsinki

Iivanainen A, Jauhiainen M, Korkiakoski L 1995 Hoitotyön käsikirja. Hygieia, Kirjayhtymä, Helsinki

Kalkas H 1982 Hoitotyön teorianmuodostuksesta. SHVK XIX, Sairaanhoitajien koulutussäätio, Helsinki

Kalkas H, Manninen K, Sammalkorpi H, Sorvettula M, Tolvanen S, Tuomaala U 1979 Hoitotyön prosessimenetelmän soveltaminen I osa. WHO: n hoitotyön kskipitkän aikavälin tutkimus – ja kehittämisohjelma. Sairaanhoidon tutkimuslaitos, Helsinki

Karhe L 2003 Teho-osaston hoitoisuusluokitus Humanistically optimised patient evaluation [Patient classification in the intensive care unit: humanistically optimised patient evaluation.] (English abstract.) Master's thesis. University of Tampere, Department of Nursing Science, Tampere

Kiikkala I 1998 Hoitotieteen perusteista ja merkityksestä käytännön hoitotyösä. Sairaanhoitaja 2: 36–38

Kiikkala I, Kokkola A, Immonen T, Ahonen J 2002 Hoitotyö asiakaslähtöisenä mielenterveyttä edistävänä toimintana. In: Kanste O, Kyngäs H, Lukkarinen H, Utriainen K (eds) Yksilöiden terveyden ja hyvinvoinnin vahvistaminen eri ympäristöissä elämänkulun kaikissa vaiheissa. VII kansallinen hoitotieteellinen konferenssi, Oulu, 91-96

Kratz C R 1993 Hoitotyön prosessi. Sairaanhoitajien koulutussäätiö, WSOY, Juva

Krause K 1983 Tutkimus ja hoitotyön kehittäminen. Tehy 22: 18–22

Krause K 1984 Hoitotyön prosessi teoriassa ja käytännössä: arvioiva tutkimus prosessiajattelun toteutumisesta. Lääkintähallitus, Helsinki

Krause K, Kiikkala I 1992 On the goals of nursing science. In: Krause K, Åstedt-Kurki P (eds) International perpectives on nursing. Tampere University Department of Nursing, Serie A 3/92, 23/34

Krause K, Salo S 1992 Teoreettinen hoitotyö. Kirjayhtymä Oy, Helsinki

LaMonica E L 1979 The nursing process. A humanistic approach. Addison Wesley, Menlo Park, CA

Latvala E, Janhonen S 1996 Potilaan selviytyminen jokapäiväisessä elämässä – psykiatrisen hoitotyön perusprosessi. [Patient's management in daily life – basic process of psychiatric nursing in hospital environment] (English summary). Hoitotiede (Journal of Nursing Science) 8: 224–232

Lauharanta J, Rotonen M 1998 Älykortti siirtää tietoa hoitoketjussa. Sairaala 1: 6–7

Lauri S 1977 Terveydenhoitajan työ 0–6-vuotiaiden lasten terveydenhoidon neuvonnassa. Mannerheimin Lastensuojeluliiton julkaisu B 24, Helsinki

Lauri S 1982a Hoitotyön prosessin kehittäminen Pohjois-Karjalan keskussairaalassa. II osa. WHO:n hoitotyön keskipitkän aikavälin tutkimus-ja kehittämisohjelman julkaisuja 10, Helsinki

Lauri S 1982b Development of the nursing process through action research. Journal of Advanced Nursing 7: 301–307

Lauri S 1984 Päätöksenteko hoitotyön prosessissa. Sairaanhoitajien koulutussäätiö, Helsinki

Lauri S 1985 Hoitotyön päätöksenteon opettaminen. Suomen Kaupunkiliiton julkaisu C 96, Helsinki

Lauri S 1990a The history of nursing research in Finland. International Journal of Nursing Studies 27(2): 169–173

Lauri S 1990b Terveydenhoitaja lapsen ja perheen hyvänolon edistäjänä. In: Krause K, Åstedt-Kurki P (eds) Hyvä olo: näkökulmia ihmisen hyvän olon edistämiseen. Sairaanhoidon tutkimuslaitoksen julkaisuja 1, Helsinki: 95–104

Lauri S 1991 Hoitotyön päätöksenteon ja tietoperustan tutkiminen: erilaisia tutkimuksellisia lähestymistapoja ja tutkimustuloksia vuosilta 1976–1991. Annales Universitatis Turkuensis C 87. Turun yliopisto. Kirjapaino Pika Oy, Turku

Lauri S (ed.) 2003 Näyttöön perustuva hoitotyö. WSOY, Helsinki

Lauri S, Eriksson E, Hupli M 1998 Hoidollinen päätöksenteko. WSOY, Kirjapainoyksikkö, Juva

Lehti T 2000 Hoitotyön kirjaaminen: seurantatutkimus Turun yliopistollisessa sairaalassa. Turun yliopistollinen keskussairaala, Turku

Lehtikunnas T, Salanterä S, Hupli M 2002 Kirjaaminen tehohoitotyössä. In: Kanste O, Kyngäs H, Lukkarinen H, Utriainen K (eds) Yksilöiden terveyden ja hyvinvoinnin vahvistaminen eri ympäristöissä elämänkulun kaikissa vaiheissa. VII kansallinen hoitotieteellinen konferenssi, Oulu: 121–125

Leino-Kilpi H 1990 Good nursing care. On what basis? Academic dissertation. Annales Universitatis Turkuensis D 49. Kirjapaino University of Turku. Pika Oy, Turku

Leino-Kilpi H, Suominen T 1998 Nursing research in Finland from 1958 to 1995. Journal of Nursing Scholarship 30(30): 363–367

Leminen A 1966 Sairaanhoidon ja sairaanhoitajan työn teoriasta. Sairaanhoidon Vuosikirja IV 1966–1967. SHKS, Helsinki

Liukkonen A 1989 Psykogeriatrisen hoitotyön toteutus mielisairaalassa. Lääkintöhallituksen julkaisuja. Tutkimukset 5/1989, Helsinki

Liukkonen A 1990 Dementoituneen potilaan perushoito laitoksessa. Academic dissertation. Annales Universitatis Turkuensis ser C 181, University of Turku, Turku

Liuksila P-R 1991 Lasten terveyskertomuslomakkeiston käyttö lapsen ja perheen terveydenhoidon toteutuksessa. Pro gradu -tutkielma. Terveydenhuollon koulutusohjelma. Hoitotieteen laitos, Turun yliopisto, Turku

Marriner A 1979 The nursing process. A scientific approach to nursing care. C V Mosby, St Louis, MI

Mattila A, Haapa-Laakso P, Tapanainen M-L, Vallimies-Patomäki M 2000 Qualification requirements for nurses, public health nurses and midwives in health care. Essential considerations related to practising health care professions. Stencils of the Ministry of Social Affairs and Health 2000:15. Ministry of Social Affairs and Health, Helsinki

Ministry of Education 2003 Available: http://www.minedu.fi/minedu/education/polytechnic.html 25 June 2003

Munnukka T 1993 Tehtävien hoidosta yksilövastuiseen hoitotyöhön. [From functional nursing to primary nursing.] (English summary.) Academic dissertation. Acta Universitatis Tamperensis, Ser. A, Vol. 375, University of Tampere, Finland

Nightingale F 1987 Sairaanhoidosta. SHKS, WSOY, Porvoo

Niskanen T, Paavilainen E, Tarkka M-T, Puura K 2002 'Varhaisen vuorovaikutuksen tukeminen lastenneuvolatyössä' – hankkeen koulutuksellisten valmiuksien ilmeneminen terveydenhoitajan viestinnässä. In: Kanste O, Kyngäs H, Lukkarinen H, Utriainen K (eds) Yksilöiden terveyden ja hyvinvoinnin vahvistaminen eri ympäristöissä elämänkulun kaikissa vaiheissa. VII kansallinen hoitotieteellinen konferenssi, Oulu: 137–140

Nissinen R 1978 Hoitoprosessin toteuttaminen ja kirjaaminen osastonhoitajien arvioimanaalue- ja keskussairaaloiden naistentautien ja sisätautien osastoilla. Sairaanhoidon Vuosikirja XV. Sairaanhoitajien koulutussäätiö, Helsinki: 101–129

Nojonen K 1990 Psykiatrisen pitkäaikaispotilaan kuntoutuminen. [The rehabilitation of a long-term patient.] (English summary.) Academic dissertation. Acta Universitatis Tamperensis, Ser. A, Vol. 283, University of Tampere, Finland

Ollikainen L 1994 Messages from the point of no return. A conceptual and empirical analysis of suicide notes left by suicide victims. Academic dissertation. Annales Universitatis Turkuensis D 164. Kirjapaino University of Turku, Pika Oy, Turku

Parviainen T 1992 Johdonmukainen eteneminen terveen- ja sairaanhoidossa. In: Parviainen T, Mölsä A, Karpov I, Kehä H (eds) Hygieia, terveyden – ja sairaanhoitajan kirjasto. Kirjayhtymä, Helsinki: 100–112

Pellikka H, Lukkarinen H, Isola A 2002 Potilaiden käsityksiä hyvästä hoidosta yhteis-päivystyksessä. In: Kanste O, Kyngäs H, Lukkarinen H, Utriainen K (eds) Yksilöiden terveyden ja hyvinvoinnin vahvistaminen eri ympäristöissä elämänkulun kaikissa vaiheissa. VII kansallinen hoitotieteellinen konferenssi, Oulu: 154–158

Perälä M-L, Hammar T, Salo A 2003 Tavoitteena asiakkaan hyvä kotiutuminen ja kotihoito In: Montin L (ed) Sairaanhoitajapäivät 2003 Luentotiivistelmät (Finnish Nursing Congress and Exhibition 03, Abstract book), Helsinki, 99

Pitkänen A, Koivunen M, Kuronen M, Mäkinen M, Oksa L, Peltonen T, Välimäki M 2003 Voidaanko osastonhoitajien varahenkilöiden johtamisvalmiuksia kehittää koulutuksen ja työnohjauksen avulla? In: Montin L (ed.) Sairaanhoitajapäivät 2003 Luentotiivistelmät (Finnish Nursing Congress and Exhibition 03, Abstract book), Helsinki, 128

Sainio C 2003 Syöpäpotilaan osallistuminen päätöksentekoon. In: Montin L (ed.) Sairaanhoitajapäivät 2003 Luentotiivistelmät (Finnish Nursing Congress and Exhibition 03, Abstract book), Helsinki, 61

Sairaalaliitto (The Hospital Association) 1979 Psykiatrinen sairauskertomus. Ohjekirja. Sairaalaliitto, Helsinki

Sairaalaliitto (The Hospital Association) 1980 Kirjallinen hoitosuunnitelma potilaan hoidon apuväline. Sairaalaliitto 2/80, Sairaalalkiito, Vammalan kirjapaino Oy, Helsinki

Sarajärvi A, Isola A 2002 Sairaanhoidon opiskelijoiden hoitotyön oppimista ohjaavat tekijät käytännön harjoittelujaksolla. In: Kanste O, Kyngäs H, Lukkarinen H, Utriainen K (eds) Yksilöiden terveyden ja hyvinvoinnin vahvistaminen eri ympäristöissä elämänkulun kaikissa vaiheissa. VII kansallinen hoitotieteellinen konferenssi, Oulu: 181–185

Saranto K 1998a Tietotekniikka kirjaamisen tulevaisuudessa. In: Hallila L (ed.) Hoitotyön kirjallinen suunnitelma. Kirjayhtymä Oy, Helsinki: 122–129

Saranto K 1998b Outcomes of education in information technology at nursing polytechnics. Health Informatics Journal 4(2): 84–91

Savolainen P, Kärki S-L 1983 Hoitotyön prosessiajattelun tausta ja perusteet. In: Sinkkonen S (ed.) Hoitotiede 1. Kustannuskiila Oy, Kuopio: 56–60

Sinkkonen S 1988 Sairaanhoidon vuosikirja. [The Yearbook of Nursing.] Sairaanhoitajien koulutussäätiö, Helsinki

Sinkkonen S 1999 Terveydenhuollon yliopistollisen koulutuksen kehityskaari ja tulevaisuuden näkymät. Tehy 18/99: 36–41

Sinkkonen S, Savolainen P 1983 Ongelmia prosessiajattelun soveltamisessa hoitotyöhön. In: Sinkkonen S (ed.) Hoitotiede. Hoitotiede 1. Kustannuskiila Oy, Kuopio: 70–71

Sorvettula M 1998 Johdatus suomalaisen hoitotyön historiaan. [Introduction to the history of Finnish nursing.] Suomen Sairaanhoitajaliitto ry, Helsinki

Suominen T, Leino-Kilpi H 1998 Review of Finnish nursing research from 1958 to 1995. Scandinavian Journal of Caring Sciences 12: 57–62

Terveydenhuollon oikeusturvakeskus [The national authority for medicolegal affairs] 2002 Terveydenhuollon ammattihenkilöiden keskusrekisteri 31.12.2002

Tuomi J 1997 Suomalainen hoitotiedekeskustelu. [The genesis of nursing and caring science in Finland.] (English summary.) Academic dissertation. University of Jyväskylä, Studies in Sport, Physical Education and Health, Jyväskylä

University of Oulu 2003 Available: http://www.oulu.fi/hoitotiede/english.htm 08 July 2003

University of Tampere 2003 Available: http://www.uta.fi/laitokset/hoito/englanti.htm. 08 July 2003

University of Turku 2003 Available: http://www.med.utu.fi/tdk/english.html. 28 July 2003

Välimäki M 1998 Self-determination in psychiatric patients. Doctoral dissertation. Annales Universitatis Turkuensis D 288, Turku University, Turku

Veteläsuo R 1967 Sairaanhoito-oppi. Sairaanhoidon koulutussäätiö. WSOY, Helsinki

World Health Organisation 1977 Development of designs in, and the documentation of the nursing process. WHO Regional Office for Europe, Copenhagen

Yura H, Walsh M B 1988 Hoitotyön kehittäminen. [The nursing process: assessing, planning, implementing, evaluating, 4 edn.] WSOY, Porvoo

Chapter 7

The Nursing Process: developments and issues in Germany

Monika Habermann

INTRODUCTION

The Nursing Process as a theoretical framework is firmly rooted in German nursing education and in legislation that governs the quality management of nursing activities. It thus constitutes a broadly unquestioned 'core of nursing'. However, as various reports from other countries throughout this volume show, there is a tacit vote taken by practitioners: two decades after its official implementation in nursing education in Germany and in spite of numerous and costly efforts in all fields of nursing to put the concept into effect, it has been realized only in fragments. The implementation of the Nursing Process, therefore, continues to be a priority on the agenda of the nursing management and nursing education. It is lauded in debates, projects and research activities as an important point of reference for further developments of the nursing profession. This is an important issue in Germany in view of the fact that nursing in this country is lagging behind international progress.

This contribution will outline some of the cornerstones of the debate focusing on the Nursing Process in several areas, such as legislation and the respective laws in different nursing fields, research and implementation projects, and theoretical considerations.

LEGISLATION AND IMPLICATIONS

What are the particular attributes of nursing, peculiar to the profession and thus accepted as 'proprium' of nursing? What are the central theories, methods and tasks that characterize the unique contribution of the profession? While lacking substantial answers, the concept of the Nursing Process seems to have answered most of the uncertainties in Germany during the 1980s. Since 1985, the Nursing Process has been defined as a basic concept of nursing education (Krankenpflegegesetz in Kurtenbach et al 1986). The German Hospital Association also mentioned the Nursing Process (or 'Krankenpflegeprozess') when it developed its ideas on quality assurance in hospitals in 1985 and recommended its use to structure nurses' work in combination with precise documentation (Grundsätze und Anforderungen an die patientenbezogene Pflegedokumentation in Krankenhäuser 1985). The Nursing Process is undoubtedly still regarded as central issue with regard to ensuring the quality of nurses' work in hospitals. Even though the term is not explicitly mentioned, it is regarded as the 'general accepted level of scientific based knowledge' in nursing and, as such, constitutes the point of departure for evaluating interventions of nurses (Sozialgesetzbuch 2004b).

In nursing homes and in home care settings, where the services rendered by nurses are central, legislation rules the Nursing Process explicitly as the framework for adequate nursing activities. Nurse managers of organizations in these two areas are accountable for the correct implementation and realization of the Nursing Process in the form of individual nursing care plans (Bekanntmachung der Gemeinsamen Grundsätze und Masstäbe zur Qualität und Qualitätssicherung einschliesslich der Verfahren zur Durchführung von Qualitätsprüfungen nach § 80 SGB XI in der ambulanten Pflege 1996).

Detailed and continually revised care plans are used for external quality controls and the lack of these plans may lead to severe sanctions (Medizinischer Dienst der Spitzenverbände der Krankenkassen 2000).

Finally, the latest developments in legislation concerning basic nursing education confirm again that the goals and procedures stated in the Nursing Process are central to quality-based vocational training in nursing (Gesetz über die Berufe in der Altenpflege 2003, Gesetz über die Berufe in der Krankenpflege und zur Änderung anderer Gesetze 2003).

The Nursing Process, as we understand it in Germany, has been described in numerous textbooks. These focus either on basic introductions, like the well-known and widely used publication of Fiechter and Meyer (1991) and other general texts on nursing (Juchli 1994, Brobst and Clark 1997, Kellnhauser et al 2000, Köther and Gnamm 2000), or focus on specialized fields like psychiatry (Stockwell 2002) and community nursing (Messer 2003). The descriptions, in principle, follow early elaborations from Yura and Walsh (1978a, 1978b), which have since been disseminated by the World Health Organisation (Weltgesundheitsorganisation Mittelfristiges Programm der Weltgesundheitsorganisation für Krankenpflege- und Hebammenwesen in Europa 1973, Ashworth et al 1987). They are based on routines of 4–6 steps, comprising the analysis and prioritizing of nursing problems, the formulation of objectives concerning care the actual nursing activities, including their documentation and, finally, their evaluation. The varying number of steps outline no substantial differences but seem to be didactically different approaches to guide practitioners. Fiechter and Meyers' (1991) more detailed six-step guidelines are widely used in Germany, possibly indicating the need for more precise instructions to help struggling practitioners. The steps of the Nursing Process are documented in care plans for which numerous formats have been developed. It is to such care plans that practitioners refer when discussing the Nursing Process, as this term seems to be unknown or meaningless to many practitioners as a theoretical concept (Höhmann et al 1996).

With regard to the nursing theories underlying the Nursing Process, most guidelines refer to concepts based on the activities of daily living as outlined by Roper, Logan and Tierney (1993) and a further differentiation by Krohwinkel (1993). Only recently has Orem's theory of 'self care' gained influence, especially in hospital settings. Acceptance of nursing diagnosis systems, as created and used in the USA (e.g. NANDA, NIC, NOC; see Chapter 1 of this volume) especially for the assessment procedure within the Nursing Process, is still not widespread in Germany.

The legal embeddedness of the Nursing Process in Germany, as mentioned above, has several implications: A growing market for guidelines, documentation systems and standard care plans based on the Nursing Process has been established (Bartsch 1995, Fickus 1995, Hattemer 1995, Hermle 1995). There have been many attempts to implement and improve process-oriented care and its respective documentation in all fields of nursing. As in other countries, however, the results of these endeavours seem to be limited. Although studies focussing on the costs of the implementation, as carried out in the UK (Mason 1999), have never been published, costs seem to be high also in Germany. Finally, since the Nursing

Process has been established with reference to international standards and as a declaration of the beginning of a new era of professionalization in Germany, most scholars do not want to alert legislators and health insurance companies to the problems surrounding the Nursing Process by subjecting it to criticism. Historical constraints, lack of professional power and scarce resources within the health care system thus constituted an important framework for debates about the Nursing Process. Some basic information will be outlined in the next section.

NURSING IN GERMANY: LAGGING BEHIND WITH REGARD TO INTERNATIONAL STANDARDS

Many characteristics of the nursing education system identify it as specifically German, both within and outside European standards (Landenberger and Ortmann 1999). Firstly, basic education for all fields of nursing has long been fragmented. Training for general, paediatric and geriatric nurses, as well as for nurses working with the disabled, is offered by different institutions, leads to different certificates and is governed by separate acts (with the exception of general nurses and paediatric nurses, who are covered by the same act). While nurses in the former two fields are trained in schools affiliated with hospitals and their training is based on the general standards for the Federal Republic, training for nurses in the latter two fields has been based on different legal regulations in the 12 states that existed in Germany when these fields were created in nursing education in the 1970s. In 2003, after much controversy and debate, a single law regulating the basic education of geriatric nurses for the whole Federal Republic was finally implemented.

With the promulgation of a range of new regulations in Germany, some progress has been made to bridge the gap between international standards and German nursing.

- It is now possible to offer integrated education.
- Within still-restrictive settings, basic nursing education can also be offered by institutions of higher education.
- The focus of nursing has been shifted: nurses care not only for individuals in actual need of medical therapy but also undertake tasks, such as health promotion and health counselling of families and individuals. Recognizing these additional responsibilities, the certificates of the former 'Krankenschwestern' and 'Krankenpfleger', therefore, now carry the extra title of 'Gesundheitsschwester' and 'Gesundheitspfleger'.
- The importance of theoretical and evidence-based work in the field of nursing is acknowledged by the increased number of hours spent on theoretical course work during the education of nurses.

Revision of the nursing acts mentioned above has still left many urgent questions unanswered. To name only a few: the basic education of general nurses is still mainly associated with hospital settings and university education will also remain the exception in the near future. A first academic degree (Bachelor) will be awarded primarily with the study of nursing man-

agement, nursing education or nursing expertise in four-year academic training courses, which have been available since the 1990s, following a basic nursing education. This is a long study period for German nurses compared to that of their international counterparts, who usually have achieved a Masters degree by that stage of their careers. Finally, the separation of the training of midwifes from that of nurses has so far been untouched by the reorganization.

There are several explanations for the difficulties experienced by German nurses to gain more professional power. Historically, nursing had been kept firmly in the grasp of religious orders, and so-called 'wild', secular nurses faced many barriers. The support for a more powerful role for nurses during the Nazi regime had been tainted by war and racial ideologies, and was consequently reversed after the war. A period of continuing fragmented and controversial representation of the profession in the public and political field followed (Haug 1995). There is still no nursing regulatory body reflecting autonomy of the profession in dealing with registration and qualification issues or sanctions. These circumstances further increased the already dominant role of the medical profession, which is also powerful in terms of numbers – an important indicator for the lack of success in professionalization efforts of nurses by international comparison (Haug 1995, Döhler 1997).

Future striving towards professional development in the nursing field might be supported by influences that favour an expansion of a well-trained nursing workforce: as in other countries, demographic changes have heightened expenditures in the health care system while at the same time lowering the number of people who contribute the social security system. Changes in the range of diseases now treatable have increased the need for well-trained nurses to provide care. As in other European countries, a critical shortage of nurses, especially in some fields of nursing, can only be partially compensated by hiring them from abroad. This shortage creates political and public pressure to develop career paths attractive to nurses. Finally, European policies with regard to nursing education have set up a framework that cannot be undermined permanently by one of the more influential countries, like Germany.

The delayed developments in nursing professionalization, as outlined above, also explain the poverty of research, especially on a high evidence base, such as randomized control studies. The establishment of university-based study courses in the 1990s has, however, created broader opportunities for research. Together with the research work of some pioneers in nursing research, the work coming from such departments is now adding to the growing body of nursing knowledge in Germany. With regard to the Nursing Process, some major projects and their results are briefly highlighted in the following section.

PROJECTS AND RESEARCH

A study focusing on the outcome of care activities based on the Nursing Process and declared as desirable in international nursing research

(Moloney and Maggs 1999) has not yet been carried out in Germany. A reasonable well-funded study focusing on the Nursing Process performed in the early 1990s is still regarded as a milestone in German nursing research. This study will be described in some detail: Commissioned by the Ministry of Health and designed as an intervention study over 3 years, Krohwinkel (1993) explored the implementation and outcome of the Nursing Process in the care of stroke patients in two hospitals. Weaknesses in the methods have been criticized in the literature, but nevertheless the exploration and analysis of nurses' performances and their documentation allowed criteria for successful nursing interventions based on process-oriented care to be outlined, such as 'visibility', 'continuity', 'holistic approach' and 'support for self-care and independency' (Krohwinkel 1993: 272). In line with a previous study (Elkeles 1988), she defined a patient-centred work organization as the decisive framework for successful implementation of process-oriented work. In view of the widely practised task-oriented routines of the time, these findings supported discourses focusing on new models of work organization in hospitals. Precise descriptions of poor performance and, in contrast, high-quality performances and their consequences for patients' rehabilitation based on this research are still used in education, and probably fostered the implementation of special stroke units in the 1990s.

Focusing on the home care sector and care for the elderly in nursing homes, Höhmann et al (1997) explored the deficits and potential of process-oriented nursing care plans. One outcome was the development of a documentation system, comprising a process-oriented nurse plan, to bridge the intersectoral and interprofessional transfer (Höhmann et al 1997). Building on this study, a second study further explored deficits in intersectoral and interprofessional coordination of care, which are known to create substantial problems with the quality of care (Höhmann et al 1998). Integrated health care minimizes communication losses at the interface of home care settings and hospital and community/residence care for the elderly, and is, therefore, actually of high priority. The central contribution of nurses towards quality-based care seems to be knowledge about care plans, their acceptance and solid documentation based on a documentation system of the Nursing Process which can be transferred between sectors.

Several studies have explored aspects of the understanding, acceptance and handling of the Nursing Process or its materialization in the form of care plans (Seidl and Walter 1988a, 1988b, Needham 1990, Lay and Brandenburg 2001, Bartholomeyczik and Morgenstern 2004). The findings are similar to those in other international research (see Chapter 1, this volume): Physical aspects of assessment, planning, documentation and evaluation of care are prominent, but communication aspects, spiritual aspects and the overall social and cultural welfare of patients are neglected. Again, in line with international findings, the first steps of the Nursing Process are better documented, while goal-setting and evaluation procedures are subsequently more poorly elaborated. Even so, based primarily on documentation analysis, it can be assumed that these results represent the realities of the actual nursing practice, since many articles by teachers and nurse managers in non-scientific nursing journals tell the same story: the full circle of the Nursing Process is not realized.

PROFESSIONAL DEBATES AND CONCLUSION

> For over 15 years, German nursing has striven to implement care plans based on the nursing process in all fields of practice. Hardly any other concept has produced so many efforts, reorientations, controversial debates and so much printed paper. In some places, nursing departments had been flooded by several introductory waves, other places are just starting projects or are about to undertake the third or fourth revision; all without leaving visible marks . . . It is the companies that produce documentation systems which have profited most, not the nurses.
>
> (Schöniger and Zegelin-Abt 1998: 305) [translated by the author]

This concluding statement, written by two nursing care scientists, draws on several contributions during the last decade criticizing the theory and practice of the Nursing Process (Andries 1991, Brodehl 1992a, 1992b, 1992c, Elsner 1995, Stratmeyer 1997, Fischbach 2001). Exploring the potential inherent message of the 'non-complicance' of German nurses, these authors point to problems with regard to the implementation of the process, which are also discussed internationally and are documented in some of the reports from other countries in this volume. Therefore, critical comments brought up in the German context will be summarized only briefly.

Firstly, as a problem-solving-process, the 'Nursing Process' is not unique but a specific application of a generally available instrument. It constitutes an instrument for structuring nursing activities that is especially useful for didactical purposes and for the support of newcomers to the practice field. This usefulness is basically not questioned. It is also conceded that a single-problem definition, like incontinence or risk of falling, and the monitoring of the outcomes of respective nursing interventions might be supported by the Nursing Process. The complexity of professional nursing is, however, seen to be reduced, when based on the Nursing Process as a central theory and instrument. It forces complex professional perceptions into simplified structures. Individual communication processes and the negotiation of possible interventions are pressed into checklist patterns that promise completeness but enhance fragmentation. The rationality of professional nursing is thus reduced to purpose-oriented acting and neglects endeavours for person-centred, holistic and individualistic strategies in nursing. As a core instrument of nursing practice, and taking into account the immense energy that is taken up by putting it into action, it might be regarded as a 'historic error of nursing' as one critical article is titled (Stratmeyer 1997).

It might add to German – and possibly international – debates, to explore the meaning of this discussion in some more detail. The fragmentation of nurses' work based on the Nursing Process is in line with medical orientations and action strategies within the mainstream of the health care system: outcomes based on analytical cause–effect strategies are the focus and the communication with patient is aimed at serving this purpose. Reports, not narratives, are required. The medical profession lacks a generally accepted comprehensive theory and acts instead as an applied science, using and producing theories within the boundaries of more or less atomistically oper-

ating subdisciplines (von Uexküll et al 1991). The Nursing Process in theory and practice fits into this medical orientation of patient care. It does not open a substantial new view on legitimizing the unique contribution of nurses in therapeutic and caring processes. At best it describes how to work in a structured way and supports a similar structured documentation.

In terms of power relations, the legal enforcement of the Nursing Process might be seen as a tool for surveillance, which enforces a paradigmatic order created and fostered by the most powerful players within the system. The propagation of the Nursing Process within the nursing profession might be read as internalization of the concept within a discipline still struggling for decisive influence to form conditions of care. If this interpretation of the discourse represents important outlines, what are the consequences? There are some suggestions: the Nursing Process may be used as a didactic approach because it ensures that basic principles for goal-oriented nursing action are learned by beginners. However, this usage should be based on, and proceeded with by continually developing theoretical conceptions that reflect the unique contribution of nursing in different fields of action. The correct handling of single techniques does not create quality nursing practice. Techniques have to be complemented by a professional response adapted to singular situations of individual patients and their particular needs. This approach needs a supporting framework: a patient-centred organizational approach in institutional and home care settings; support for advanced nurse practitioners to emancipate themselves from checklist-focused structures, and allow them to set reasonable priorities and develop individualized care plans accordingly; and, last but not least, a scholarly debate on nursing care, which should address the growing need for professional care in the society, based on patient-centred theories and derived instruments. Such a framework could supply a solid strategy in the search for the 'proprium' of nursing, which has not emerged as yet.

REFERENCES

Andries A 1991 Probleme mit der Pflegeplanung. Die Schwester, Der Pfleger 30(9): 812–815

Ashworth P, Björn A, Dechanoz G et al 1987 People's need for nursing care: a European study. World Health Organisation Regional Office for Europe, Copenhagen

Bartholomeyczik S, Morgenstern M 2004 Qualtiätsdimensionen in der Pflegedokumentation. Pflege 17(1): 187–196

Bartsch S 1995 Standardpflegeplan bei chronischer Niereninsuffizienz. Die Schwester, Der Pfleger 34(12): 1091–1102

Bekanntmachung der Gemeinsamen Grundsätze und Maßstäbe zur Qualität und Qualitätssicherung einschließlich der Verfahren zur Durchführung von Qualitätsprüfungen nach § 80 SGB XI in der ambulanten Pflege 1996 as Amendment to the LongTerm Care Act; Bundesanzeiger 48, Berlin

Brobst R, Clark C 1997 Der Pflegeprozeß in der Praxis Huber, Bern

Brodehl R 1992a Pflegeprozess: Utopie oder gangbarer Weg? (Teil I) Die Schwester, Der Pfleger 31(4): 318–323

Brodehl R 1992b Pflegeprozess: Utopie oder gangbarer Weg? (Teil II) Die Schwester, Der Pfleger 31(6): 556–561

Brodehl R 1992c Pflegeprozess: Utopie oder gangbarer Weg? (Teil III) Die Schwester, Der Pfleger 31(7): 675–681

Döhler M 1997 Die Regulierung von Professionsgrenzen. Struktur und Entwicklungsdynamik von Gesundheitsberufen im internationalen Vergleich. Campus, Frankfurt

Elkeles J 1988 Arbeitsorganisation in der Krankenpflege – Zur Kritik der Funktionspflege. Köln

Elsner B 1995 Der Pflegeprozess erfüllt die Hoffungen nicht. Die Schwester, Der Pfleger 34(2): 91–96

Fickus P 1995 Standardpflegeplan zur postoperativen Pflege von Patienten mit Aortocoronarem Venenbypass. Die Schwester/Der Pfleger 34(7): 687–695

Fiechter V, Meyer M 1991 Pflegeplanung eine Anleitung für die Praxis. Recom, Basel

Fischbach A 2001 Vom Ende des Pflegeprozesses. Die Schwester, Der Pfleger 40: 173–175

Gesetz über die Berufe in der Altenpflege 2003 In Bundesgesetzblatt Teil I, 44, ausgegeben zu Bonn am 4: 1691–1696

Gesetz über die Berufe in der Krankenpflege und zur Änderung anderer Gesetze. Bundesgesetzblatt I 2003: 1442–1456

Grundsätze zur Anforderung an die patientenbezogene Pflegedokumentation in Krankenhäuser 1985. Die Schwester, Der Pfleger 24(8): 663

Haug K 1995 Professionaliserungsstrategien, Durchsetzungspotentiale und Arbeitsteilung. Eine Untersuchung bei deutschen und englischen Pflegekräften. Research Unit Public Health Policy Wissenschaftszentrum, Berlin

Hattemer M 1995 Standardpflegplan 'Parkinsonsche Krankheit'. Die Schwester, Der Pfleger 34(6): 496–508

Hermle V 1995 Standardpflegeplan bei Neurodermitis – mit individuellem Pflegeplan. Die Schwester, Der Pfleger 35(6): 515–525

Höhmann U, Weinrich H, Gätschenberger G 1996 Die Bedeutung des Pflegeplanes für die Qualitätssicherung in der Pflege (Reihe: Forschungsberichte Sozialforschung Bd. 261). Bundesministerium für Sozialordnung, Bonn

Höhmann U, Weinrich H Gätschenberger G 1997 Neues Dokumentationssystem zur vereinfachten patientenbezogenen Umsetzung des Pflegeprozesses in ambulanter und stationärer Langzeitpflege Pflege 3: 157–164

Höhmann U, Müller-Mundt G, Schulz B 1998 Qualität durch Kooperation – Gesundheitsdienste in der Vernetzung. Mabuse, Frankfurt a M

Juchli L 1994 Pflege, Praxis und Theorie der Gesundheits- und Krankenpflege. 7. Auflage, Thieme, Stuttgart

Kellnhauser E, Schewior-Popp S, Geißner U, Sitzmann F, Gümmer M, Ullrich L 2000 Pflege. Thieme, Stuttgart

Köther I, Gnamm E 2000 Altenpflege in Ausbildung und Praxis, 4th edn. Thieme, Stuttgart

Kurtenbach H, Golombek G, Siebers H 1986 Krankenpflegegesetz. Kohlhammer, Stuttgart

Krohwinkel M 1993 Der Pflegeprozess am Beispiel von Apoplexiekranken. Eine Studie zur Erfassung und Entwicklung ganzheitlich-rehabilitierender Prozeßpflege. Nomos Verlag, Baden-Baden

Landenberger M, Ortmann J 1999 Pflegeberufe im europäischen Vergleich. Expertise der Berufs- und Ausbildungssituation in der Alten-, Kranken- und Behindertenpflege. BBJ Verlag, Berlin

Lay R, Brandenburg H 2001 Pflegeplanung abschaffen? Überlegungen aus wissenschaftlicher Sicht. Die Schwester, Der Pfleger 40: 938–942

Mason C 1999 Guide to practice or 'load of rubbish'? The influence of care plans on nursing practice in five clinical areas in Northern Ireland. Journal of Advanced Nursing 29(2): 380–387

Medizinischer Dienst der Spitzenverbände der Krankenkassen MDK-Anleitung zur Prüfung der Qualität nach § 80 SGB XI in der Ambulanten Pflege 2000. Online. Available: http://www.vincentz.net/download/MDK-Anleitung-am-07062000.pdf 4 November 2004

Messer B 2003 Tägliche Pflegeplanung in der ambulanten Pflege. Beispiele und Lösungen. Schlütersche, Hannover

Moloney R, Maggs C A 1999 A systematic review of the relationships between written manual nursing care planning, record keeping and patient outcomes. Journal of Advanced Nursing 30 (1): 51–57

Needham I 1990 Ansichten und Meinungen zum Pflegeprozeß: Eine hermeneutische Untersuchung von Aussagen in Fachschriftenartikeln. Pflege 3(1): 59–67

Roper N, Logan WW, Tierney A 1993 Die Elemente der Krankenpflege. Ein Pflegemodell das auf einem Lebensmodell beruht. Recom, Basel

Schöniger U, Zegelin-Abt A 1998 Hat der Pflegeprozess ausgedient? Die Schwester, Der Pfleger 37(4): 305–310

Seidl E, Walter I 1988a Verbessert die Pflegeplanung die Praxis? Untersuchung von 100 Pflegedokumentationen. Pflege 1(1): 50–56

Seidl E, Walter I 1988b Verbessert die Pflegeplanung die Praxis? Untersuchung von 100 Pflegedokumentationen. Pflege 1(2): 104–111

Sozialgesetzbuch Elftes Buch Soziale Pflegeversicherung 2004a In: Krankenhausrecht, 12th edn. Deutsche Krankenhausgesellschaft, Düsseldorf: 495–570

Sozialgesetzbuch Fünftes Buch Gesetzliche Krankenversicherung 2004b In: Krankenhausrecht, 12th edn. Deutsche Krankenhausgesellschaft, Düsseldorf: 229–492

Stratmeyer P 1997 Ein historischer Irrtum der Pflege. Plädoyer für einen kritisch-distanzierten Umgang mit dem Pflegeprozess. Dr. med. Mabuse 106: 34–38

Stockwell F 2002 Der Pflegeprozess in der psychiatrischen Pflege. Huber, Bern

Uexküll T von, Wesiack W 1991 Theorie der Humanmedizin. Grundlagen ärztlichen Denkens und Handelns. Urban & Schwarzenberg. München

Weltgesundheitsorganisation Mittelfristiges Programm der Weltgesundheitsorganisation (WGO) für Krankenpflege- und Hebammenwesen in Europa 1973 Deutsche Krankenpflegezeitschrift 7: 15–16

Yura H, Walsh M B 1978a The nursing process: assessing, planning, implementing, evaluating. Appleton Century Crofts, New York

Yura H, Walsh M B 1978b Human needs and the nursing process. Appleton Century Crofts, New York

Chapter **8**

The Nursing Process in Australia

Bev Taylor and Chris Game

INTRODUCTION

In Australia, it seems that the Nursing Process has gone through phases of resistance, acceptance and institutionalization. From the original resistance to it in clinical areas in the 1970s, through a begrudging acceptance of it in the 1980s, the Nursing Process has become so familiar as to become institutionalized, by being reduced to its barest functional level. The present-day status of the Nursing Process is that it is being used in most clinical areas, but it has been made more palatable and manageable by being used mainly as the structure of nursing care plan checklists.

The Nursing Process has also attracted minimal attention in the nursing literature, possibly owing to the fact that it was introduced into Australia at a time when nurses were not engaging actively in research, tertiary studies and scholarship. Therefore, a search of the literature revealed little to assist in the compilation of this chapter.

Searching with the keywords 'Nursing Process', 'process' and 'Australia', six articles were located in CINAHL, all published before 1997. A Medline search located 31 articles, all pre-1997, few of which were suitable for this chapter. The Fulltext Nursing Database located 36 articles, the majority of which were not Australian. Ebsco Host – Health/Nursing Academic literature and Ovid databases located some full text articles relating indirectly and obliquely to the Nursing Process (Duffield et al 1996, Mitchell 1997, Usher 1998, Stockdale 2000, Taylor 2000, McAllister 2003), in that they related to caring in practice and nursing care delivery systems. A manual library search found some early articles about the Nursing Process (Watson 1982, Cook 1983, Yuen 1986, Graunke 1988, Paech and Oreo 1994).

Approaches to the two main national professional organizations, the Royal College of Nursing Australia, and the College of Nursing, formerly the College of Nursing, New South Wales, indicated that they did not have specific archival documents and publications relating to the Nursing Process. Therefore, the historical description for this chapter is reliant on the first-hand account of Ms Chris Game, a nurse of 38 years experience, with a strong interest in history, who offers personal experiential information as a coauthor.

DEFINITIONS OF THE NURSING PROCESS

Initially, in the Australian nursing profession, the Nursing Process was defined simply as a problem-solving approach, involving the phases of assessing, planning, implementing and evaluating nursing care. By the end of the 1970s, Australia progressed, as part of the international movement, to couching generalized nursing problems in the language of nursing diagnoses (Crisp and Taylor 2001) according to the format of the North American Nursing Diagnosis Association (NANDA).

A review of the available Australian literature reveals that the Nursing Process was defined originally as the assessment, planning, implementation and evaluation of nursing care, and the four steps had almost become an international mantra amongst nurses, to the extent that some later articles did not even bother to define the Nursing Process (Cook 1983, Yuen 1986,

O'Brien 1988). By the early 1980s, there was a general feeling among Australian nurses that the Nursing Process had been 'done to death' and some nurses might have considered its 'demise highly desirable', although other nurses recognized that the Nursing Process had the potential to widen the dimensions of nursing practice and further develop its professional growth (Cook 1983: 40). By the end of the 1980s and into the early 1990s, references to the Nursing Process defined it as a five-step approach with the specific inclusion of diagnosis after the assessment phase (Doheny et al 1987, Paech and Oreo 1994).

NATIONAL REGULATIONS

While the use of the Nursing Process is not *enforced* nationally as such, in that it is not absolutely compulsory in every facet of Australian nursing, it is highly recommended in nursing practice and education. For example, in national undergraduate Bachelor of Nursing programmes, universities are responsible for educating graduates, who are capable of reaching the Australian Nursing Council Incorporated (ANCI) standards or competencies for a registered nurse. These competencies require Bachelor of Nursing programmes to teach the Nursing Process and to assess the students' implementation of it in clinical practice. Therefore, there is a level of enforcement by state registration boards for first-level graduates, so they achieve a satisfactory grounding in the Nursing Process to use as graduates.

The Nursing Process is also enshrined within the audits of nursing documentation processes in the accreditation processes of hospitals. If a hospital is not using a valid method of documenting nursing care, they will not achieve accreditation. Traditionally, the accepted method of nursing care documentation is based on the Nursing Process.

The mid-point between the university education system and the hospital accreditation processes is the profession of nursing. It is interesting that, by the late 1980s, the specialist colleges, such as the critical care nurses' college, the operating nurses' group and community nurses' groups, were professional groups endorsing the utilization of the Nursing Process. Therefore, the Nursing Process was enforced by education and workplace requirements, and the profession was constantly adapting it to their particular area of specialty. For clinical nurses, it was a process that was practical and plausible to use, because nursing care is best implemented when a time of assessment and planning has elapsed and, reasonably, care is improved through constant and careful evaluation.

HISTORY

In Australia, the first undergraduate programmes to prepare nurses for registration outside the hospital setting and the old apprenticeship programme commenced in 1974, as a result of funding from the Commonwealth Tertiary Education Commission (CTEC). It was at that time also that the Nursing Process came from America to Australia. The Executive Director of the College, Pat Slater, had undertaken a Masters degree in the USA. Whilst in the USA, she decided to promote tertiary basis for the preparation of the registered nurse in Australia, and on her return, she introduced the Nursing Process through the Royal College of Nursing, Australia (RCAN), which was then the College of Nursing, Australia (CNA). The first non-hospital course was a pilot programme undertaken at the CNA in Melbourne. The first intake commenced in 1974 with a cohort of 20 students.

The Nursing Process was an easy process to use. The significant point about the Nursing Process was that it also formed the basis of the competencies assessment of each year in the initial CNA tertiary nursing programme. For example, when students went into clinical practice placements, they not only had to perform and gain a pass evaluation in the traditional clinical hands-on nursing skills, such as bed making, dressings, enemas, intravenous apparatus and so on, but they also, as part of their daily assessment, developed nursing care plans using the Nursing Process for patients with whom they were assigned.

CNA educators also used the Nursing Process to develop the assessment tool, which was used as the formal and summative assessment for each student in each year. The particular assessment process was developed in consultation with Monash University, in the School of Education, where there was a research group appointed by the CTEC to oversee the evaluation of this pilot programme. This was because the Commonwealth wanted feedback on whether the programme would work and if they were prepared to fund other states in tertiary nursing programmes. History shows us that this is what happened.

Following the successful implementation of the pilot Diploma in Nursing at the CNA in 1974, and the releasing of the Stage 1 report on the evaluation of the first cohort in 1977, the Commonwealth approved the establishment of further Diploma in Nursing programmes at Cumberland College in Sydney, Queensland Institute of Technology in Brisbane, West Australian College of Advanced Education (CAE) in Perth and Sturt CAE in South Australia.

The nursing profession began to agitate for more diploma programmes and to scale down the intakes for hospital-based courses, with a view to a total transfer no later than 1982. This move followed the successful second National Conference on the Goals in Nursing Education in 1978. The Commonwealth commissioned a review of nursing education in the higher education sector chaired by Dr Sidney Sax, and this report was published in 1978. The report, whilst praising the existing programmes, actually counselled the Commonwealth against taking on the full burden of the cost of nursing education and instead recommended a continuation of hospital-based courses, with only a limited number of Diploma in Nursing courses in the higher education sector. In addition, Sax recommended that these nursing courses should remain at the level of undergraduate diploma and he actively recommended against the establishment of degree studies for nurses.

At the Annual National Conference of the CNA immediately following the release of the Sax Report, members of the profession present in Adelaide 'took to the streets' in demonstration against the findings of the Sax Report. This demonstration culminated in a ritual burning of the Sax Report in a bedpan and made front-page news in all states. What then followed was a number of years during which nurse leaders kept up the pressure on both state and Commonwealth governments to advance the cause of the transfer of nursing education. This culminated in a move by the New South Wales Government to decree that all hospital-based certificate programmes in nursing would cease to have intakes from the beginning of 1985 and from that date these programmes would transfer to the CAEs. Whilst this was revolutionary and caused a domino effect throughout all other states and territories, it was not until 1992 that the final state, Queensland, completed the transfer.

Even though the Nursing Process was part of the new move into tertiary education, it would be fair to say that the majority of nurses who were on the teaching staff at the time felt: 'Ah, yeah, it's more of American bunkum that we are going through'. The basis for this attitude was that the CNA students were already different from any other nursing student in the clinical agencies. The CNA was using clinical agencies that were still running hospital-based programmes. Therefore, CNA students were working alongside students who were working in apprenticeship programmes. CNA nurses were already conspicuous, because their uniforms were different, and they came into placement settings with a clinical teacher who remained with them at all times in their clinical practice, while practising skills, implementing and documenting patient care. That was an unusual system for apprenticeship students, who worked for a wage according to the requirements of the health care setting.

From 1978, it took 5–6 years for the tertiary-based nurses in hospitals and the profession at large slowly to accept and establish the Nursing Process. Many clinical nurses in hospitals ridiculed the Nursing Process, because they saw it as nothing more than yet another layer of documentation they had to complete. Ultimately, when it was explained, clinical nurses could see that the Nursing Process was going to help in the delivery of nursing care. Publications around that time (Watson 1982, Cook 1983) and since (Graunke 1988, O'Brien 1988) have encouraged nurses to use the Nursing Process.

It was not until 1982 that the accreditation guide changed and made it a requirement of the audit that there be a clear definition of nursing care plans. The accreditation teams did not use the words 'Nursing Process' but they dictated a clear definition of a nursing care plan, thus revealing the degree to which the Nursing Process had infiltrated the Australian health care system. The national standards process infiltrated the culture of nursing, but the trigger for the Nursing Process and its utilization in Australia was the development of Australia-wide tertiary education programmes for nursing. It is doubtful that the Nursing Process would have been as successfully implemented or entrenched, if it had not been for the move of nursing education away from the hospital apprenticeship programmes into the tertiary sector. By 1980, as experienced by the teachers involved, it seemed that every hospital in the State of Victoria in Australia, to a lesser or greater extent, had taken up use of the Nursing Process, and it was required to form the basis of documentation for nursing care.

Present-day literature relating to the Nursing Process and nursing diagnoses tends to focus mainly on its limitations and perceived shortcomings

(Taylor 2000, McAlister 2003). For example, Taylor (2000) claims that too little attention has been given to understanding and transmitting problem-solving knowledge and skills, and McAlister (2003) advocates changing the focus of patient care from problem-focused to solution-focused nursing. The present-day status of the Nursing Process is that it is being used in most clinical areas, such as surgical and medical wards, but in settings where there is an emphasis on getting the work done within the available resource allocations because of lack of staff, it has been reduced to practical check-lists that require little more than a tick in a column as tokenistic problem solving within minimal practice requirements.

IMPACT AND PROBLEMS

Problems associated with the Nursing Process in Australia are only frag-mentarily reported in the literature as stated above. Thus, the following out-lines of problems follow assumptions and experiences as they are part of common nursing discourses and experiences.

The major impact of the Nursing Process has been that it now underpins nursing practice within clinical environment and it also underpins the teaching of nursing to neophyte groups. In Australia, it is not possible to undertake a Bachelor of Nursing programme without learning about the Nursing Process: each programme throughout the country needs to adhere to the ANCI standards for competency of a first-level practising graduate nurse. These standards include a working application and knowledge of the Nursing Process.

A problem associated with the Nursing Process was that it was originally designed as a holistic approach, but it was thwarted by problems because nurses tended initially to concentrate on the medical diagnosis and treatment of the patient, and tried to reflect all of the nursing care in terms of the medical management. With the advent of NANDA, nurses had specific nursing diagnostic groups and nursing diagnoses within those groups so they were then able to embrace fully the holistic nature of nursing assessment. Another problem with the Nursing Process has been the tendency to simplify its use to a checklist. The Nursing Process was designed to be a textual document, to be written in words of more than one syllable, stating the patient's problem, and the planning and implementation phases of care to alleviate that problem. Even though many hospitals now implement the Nursing Process and nursing care plans, one of the main problems is that, once it became regimented, nurses immediately tried to find shortcuts to establish and maintain it. Consequently, there exist in many clinical practice areas, checklists with the barest details and a generic approach to care. The Nursing Process was established because nurses were concerned that nursing was becoming too task-oriented and they needed a holistic way of describing nursing care. Australian nursing has now come full circle and clinical areas use nursing care plans reduced to a set of checklists, thus running the risk of reducing the Nursing Process to task orientation again.

Another issue has arisen with the storage of the nursing care plans. Originally, the nursing care plan was readily available for nurses who were actually delivering the care, so that they had a constant check on a patient's progress. The care plan would be at the patient's bedside, so that nurses could come along and pick up the care plan, see what was planned for that patient, and then talk to that patient about the delivery and effects of care. Increasingly, and possibly because of the changes in the privacy laws and the legal system regarding privacy and confidentiality, there has been a move over the past 15 years, to remove the nursing care plans from the patients' bedsides. A positive view as nurses experience changes in technology is, therefore, that we may reach a point where we have a computer terminal beside every patient, and with the use of password protection, the care plans will return to the bedside, thus enhancing a continued actualization of the plan.

Findings in the literature also focus on problems associated with the Nursing Process. Paech and Oreo (1994) argue that the process does not assist nurses in how to manage each phase, that it stifles intuition and that it reduces care to mechanistic problem-solving. Mostafanejad (1995: 38) concluded that the Nursing Process was 'more hype than help' for nurses who 'resent being expected to do more work, while staff numbers and resources remain the same or are reduced'. Whatever the problems, it is very difficult to argue effectively against a problem-solving system that has as its prime intention the delivery and documentation of quality nursing care, even if its impact has brought with it localized problems in underresourced work settings.

THE NURSING PROCESS AND FIELDS OF NURSING

The Nursing Process is used in all fields of nursing, but it is mostly practised in the traditional general nursing, medical–surgical areas of nursing, for adults and children. Any general ward in a hospital will have nursing care plans hanging on either the end of the patient's bed, or stored in the folders containing their history. The patient's history refers to the folder where nursing care plan resides or is kept for safe keeping, and this folder also contains the clinical documents. The majority of specialist areas have nursing care plans based on the Nursing Process, because NANDA nursing diagnostic groups are still being used for teaching of the Nursing Process and in clinical practice, as nursing diagnoses exist for the total human condition. There are elements of the Nursing Process in community nursing, aged care nursing, critical care or high dependency, and operating room nursing. These are used to a larger extent in some areas and to a lesser extent in others.

Although the Nursing Process is a fundamental component in any Bachelor of Nursing programme, it is losing its importance in postgraduate research, and in clinical nursing studies at postgraduate level. This phenomenon may be due to the change in the nature of postgraduate nursing, in that the first specialist courses, such as orthopaedic and oncology nursing certificates, etc., were medically oriented. With the increase and strengthening of nursing research, most of those clinical postgraduate courses are becoming more research based. Also, there is a perception that the Nursing Process fits best with novices, who are learning how to provide nursing care.

Postgraduates with years of nursing experience, focus instead on areas of interest to them in advanced nursing practice.

THEORIES UNDERLYING THE NURSING PROCESS

There has been no attempt in Australia to tie the Nursing Process to one nursing model or theory. The authors can only speculate on the reasons for this, given the lack of research and having lived through the changes themselves. They suspect that the refusal to use a specific model or theory had to do with the attitudes towards 'imported' nursing models and theories in general, and the begrudging acceptance of the Nursing Process itself. The prevailing attitude in the early 1970s in clinical areas and hospital nursing schools was: 'We are nursing well already. We do not need these ideas to make our practice better'. At the time that the Nursing Process was introduced to Australia, there were few nurses with higher degrees and those who had attained these degrees tended to study in discipline areas outside nursing. Nurses with higher degrees in nursing often procured them in America and brought back innovative ideas, such as the Nursing Process and associated models and theories, to a population of nurses working in practice, education and administration, who were only just coming to terms with the fact that tertiary nursing was becoming a reality. Unless nurses had been exposed to nursing scholarship and research in their studies, or in their work experiences overseas, they were mainly unaware of the vast amounts of scholarly and research work filling discipline-specific books and journal articles.

If one model was acceptable to Australian nurses in those early days of the use of the Nursing Process, it was the Activities of Daily Living (ADL) approach of Roper, Logan and Tierney (1980). This model did not have the lengthy information of the American models and theories, perceived as esoteric. Rather it was an infinitely practical and a characteristically 'no-frills' British approach to working out how to deliver person-centred nursing care. As tertiary nursing became established in Australia, more and more nurses became aware of the Nursing Process, and nursing models and theories. Since then a vast array of models (Peplau 1952, Orlando 1961, Rogers 1970, Leininger 1979, Orem 1987) has been connected to the Nursing Process, depending on the needs of the particular nursing areas, and the propensities of the nurses in those areas to apply them willingly and usefully.

THE NURSING DIAGNOSES SYSTEM

The nursing diagnoses system used in Australia, imported originally from America and Canada, has taken root and is known nationally as 'NANDA'. The beginning of the NANDA movement was tied into the growing sense of professional identity and scholarliness, when Australian nurses acknowledged that nursing has its own body of knowledge, which can be expressed through nursing models, theories, research and service delivery systems, such as the Nursing Process, and nursing diagnoses.

Initially, some nursing diagnoses may have been consistent with medical diagnoses. However, in general, this is not necessarily so because nurses were attempting to look at the whole person and not just the disease. For example, in the late 1970s and early 1980s, there were some memorable inter-actions between student nurses and doctors and medical students in the clinical agencies, when the doctors would laughingly ask: 'So what's your nursing diagnosis nurse?' The nurse would reply with nursing diagnostic statements, such as 'Isolation, due to the fact that the person has been placed in the hospital far away from home and has no support structures'. There-fore, the isolation was a nursing diagnosis. The doctors could not believe that nurses were interested in that component of the patient.

As time has passed, there has been a growing critique of nursing diag-noses, as they relate to the overall Nursing Process. Nursing diagnoses have been criticized for being overly wordy, rigid and reductionist, with biomedical overtones, and of being 'imported' unnecessarily into the Australian context, as a time-consuming process for already busy practi-tioners (Masso 1990, Lawler 1991, Owen and Kelly 1991, Prideau 1991).

COMPUTERIZATION

On the whole, computers are not in widespread use at patients' bedsides, but they are being used increasingly at nurses' desks and in high-dependency and critical care areas, where one-to-one nursing is practised.

The usefulness of computerized documentation is the way forward for all fields of nursing, once real and imagined constraints can be overcome, such as a general cringe against all things technological, a lack of education and training in using computers, and phasing in of computer-based docu-ments concomitant with a decrease in paper-based communication. These processes imply the need for health care agencies to make a commitment to computerization in their budget projections and gradually to build staff con-fidence in electronic communication systems.

Darbyshire (2000) researched the practice politics of computerized patient information systems (CPIS) using focus group interviews. When he explored the attitudes of Australian nurses and midwives towards their experiences of using CPIS, he found that nurses were dissatisfied with their use because CPIS are perceived as being 'dumped' on them from the top of the hierar-chy and that these systems are about information management, not clinical information. In considering the findings, Darbyshire (2000: 17) concluded that, when forced to use CPIS, what nurses 'seem to do is to "make the best of a bad job" by trying to adapt and modify CPIS, either explicitly or sur-reptitiously in order to make them fit nurses' clinical reality'. The adjust-ment to the clinical reality of computerized systems is akin to what happened with the Nursing Process, in that nurses simply reacted to a top-down directive by making it suit their purposes. While this may on the surface seem like passive resistance, it nevertheless has resulted in an initial begrudging acceptance, which can be modified over time, as knowledge, skills and confidence increase.

RESEARCH

Australian published research into the Nursing Process has been minimal (Mostafanejad 1995, Duffield et al 1996, O'Connell 1998, 2000). This is not to deny the possibility that other research may have been done in hospital settings and health care facilities, such as community departments and aged care services, which have not been published via academic refereed processes. It is highly likely that research documents exist within the archives of hospital libraries, and in the office files of hospital and health care research departments, as the use of the Nursing Process has been monitored through quality assurance procedures to gain and maintain hospital accreditation. Unfortunately, tracking down these research projects as data sources would be a highly costly and difficult project, given the need to access thousands of hospital and health care facility sites nationwide, having gained ethical approval for the search through just as many ethics committees. A research project of this magnitude is beyond the scope of the requirements for writing this chapter, but it could be a potential research area with adequate funding.

Using an anonymous survey of nurses (n86) in the mid-west of Western Australia, Mostafanejad (1995: 36) found evidence to answer the question: 'Nursing Process – more hype than help?' The research surveyed three hospitals. Respondents had been 46 registered nurses (3 years preparation for practice, with full registration), 36 enrolled nurses (1 year preparation for practice, enrolled with restricted accountabilities) and 4 nurses who did not indicate their professional status. The project was undertaken because the Nursing Process had been gradually introduced into the Western Australian nursing curricula from 1975, and doubt had been raised as to its relevance and usefulness. The researchers were also responding to criticisms of the Nursing Process in the literature (Bowman et al 1983; Nicklin 1984, McHugh 1987, cited in Mostafanejad 1995, Lewis 1988).

The researchers surveyed nurses in one hospital (n63) using the Nursing Process and nurses in two hospitals (n23) not using it, to 'see whether its use influenced the attitude of the nurses towards the Nursing Process' (Mostafanejad 1995: 37). The questionnaire (Bowman et al 1983) had 20 items – 10 positive, 10 negative – each allocated a score of one to five, with five reflecting a very positive attitude and one a very negative attitude. Therefore, 100 denoted the highest score (most positive), 20 denoted the lowest score (most negative) and 60 denoted a neutral score. Thus, a score above 60 was regarded as positive and below 60 was regarded as negative.

The results were interesting in that the 'mean attitude score for all three hospitals combined was 59.79 which falls in the neutral range' and that the score for the hospital using the Nursing Process was 5.99 points lower than the two hospitals where it was not used (Mostafanejad 1995: 37). When the researchers compared these scores with three other projects using the same questionnaire, they found the West Australian scores to be much lower than UK nurses (Bowman et al 1983) and significantly lower than findings in New Zealand. In looking into why the scores were much lower in Western Australia, the researchers theorized that Western Australian nurses were of an older age group and that 'older nurses have less enthusiasm for the Nursing Process' as 'the oldest nurse scored 10 points lower than the youngest' (Mostafanejad 1995: 37). The researchers concluded that:

> nurses in this survey who use the Nursing Process resent being expected to do more work, while staff numbers and resources remain the same or

are reduced. As long as 'mass production' working conditions exist in the health care system, nurses can only cope with their work load by being as mechanically efficient as possible and by using assembly line-task oriented-methods in order to meet the basic physical needs of patients.

(Mostafancejad, 1995: 38)

Duffield et al. (1996: 334) explored the research question: 'Do clinical nurse specialists and managers believe that the provision of quality care is important?' They explain that, in 1986, the positions of clinical nurse specialist and nurse unit manager were introduced into New South Wales (NSW), Australia (Duffield 1996: 334). The nurse unit manager role was focused on managing the ward or unit, and the clinical nurse specialist role was concerned with clinical expertise and leadership. Given the prevailing climate of economic rationalism, the researchers were interested in the competencies expected of nurses in these positions and how the roles provided quality care. The researchers defined competence as 'the ability of the individual to fulfil her or his role effectively and/or expertly' (Report to the Australasian Nurse Registering Authorities' Conference 1990, in Duffield et al 1996: 335).

A separate study was designed for each cohort; the study for the nurse unit managers was conducted first, and the nurse specialists' study was undertaken a year later. Duffield et al (1996: 335) report that:

In the nurse unit manager study, 412 questionnaires were distributed to 34 hospitals and 318 were returned giving an acceptable response rate of 77%. A total of 958 questionnaires were distributed to clinical nurse specialists in the hospitals selected. Unfortunately, despite using the same strategies for distribution, there were only 373 complete responses returned, achieving a response rate of 39%.

The research process involved piloting a two-part instrument with the nurse unit managers, the first part being a 23-item demographic questionnaire relating to employment data, education and career paths, and the second part dealt with functional management, staff management, patient care management and leadership. A six-point Likert scale was used for subjects' responses, with six indicating strong agreement and one indicating strong disagreement with the item. The original instrument was adapted for clinical nurse specialists in the second study.

Analysis was by the calculation of mean and standard deviation for each competency from the Likert scale responses for both samples. The four main aspects reflecting the items were legal aspects, care delivery, care management and communication. In care delivery specifically, the researchers noted 'using the Nursing Process' was low for both groups and they surmised that this 'may reflect the commonly acknowledged lack of popularity for the Nursing Process or newer approaches to planning care, such as critical paths' (Duffield et al 1996: 337). Although this study was not centering on the Nursing Process *per se*, but rather the role competencies of nurse unit managers and clinical nurse specialists, it nevertheless uncovered lack of support for the Nursing Process at high leadership levels in clinical nursing management and practice in NSW at that time, a situation which has arguably not changed to the present day.

O'Connell (1998) investigated claims that there are negative attitudes towards the Nursing Process and that it is of little real use for nursing practice. She used a grounded theory approach 'to describe and theorise about the way in which the Nursing Process was used in clinical settings' (O'Connell 1998: 23), in order to identify contextual factors to account for the possible difficulties in the application of the Nursing Process in nursing practice. In her research abstract, O'Connell (1998: 22) summarised the research approach thus:

> Data were obtained from semi-structured interviews with predominantly nurse clinicians ($n = 27$), participant field observations of nurse clinicians, and in-depth audits of patient records. Textual data were managed using NUD.IST and analysed using constant comparative method. Data generation and analysis proceeded simultaneously using open ended coding, theoretical coding, and selective coding techniques until saturation was achieved.

She found that nurses experienced the basic social problem of being in a state of unknowing, linked to 'the existence of a fragmented and inconsistent method of determining and communicating patient care and work conditions of immense change and uncertainty' (O'Connell 1998: 22). This meant that nurses did their best to work in less than ideal conditions, but they feared that patient care was being compromised, because of setting constraints, such as difficulties with using the Nursing Process during nursing admission assessments, when little more than the medical diagnosis and treatment was known. This resulted in a focus on physical care, as insufficient time had elapsed in which to get to know patients on social and emotional levels. Added to this, nurses reported lack of continuity in caring owing to staffing problems and a fluctuating and uncertain working context, all of which added to their sense of unknowing. In concluding the report, O'Connell (1998: 31) commented that:

> the findings of this study revealed that the problem solving approach to care, as explicated by the Nursing Process, was difficult to achieve and nurses experienced a basic social problem of being in a state of 'unknowing' . . . The clinical conditions in acute care settings are non conducive to the implementation of a problem solving approach to care such as the Nursing Process. Wherever the problems lie, negotiating solutions remains a professional challenge. If these findings are representative of what is widely practised, there is a need to review the utility of using the Nursing Process in its current form; as the a priori assumptions of the Nursing Process, enhancing communication and professionalism, were not clinically evident.

In later research, O'Connell used a grounded theory approach to explore the process that nurses used to determine, deliver and communicate patient care in acute care settings. She used the same methods as the 1998 research and the findings revealed 'a number of factors that hindered nurses from using the Nursing Process in its current form (O'Connell 2000: 32). The complexity of nursing care was reflected in the nurses' descriptions of their need for 'putting the pieces together', by drawing on 'the known' aspects of a patient during handover, in constantly collecting, combining and pooling information, and in checking, integrating and sustaining patient information during a working shift (O'Connell 2000: 32). To minimize uncertainty, nurses adapted their work practices, took control of the care, organized doctors, and backed up each other when minor errors occurred (O'Connell 2000: 32).

Even with all of these strategies for managing hindering factors, nurses expressed professional disillusionment as a consequence of working through obscurity and uncertainty. As O'Connell (2000: 37) explained, nurses

> were dissatisfied with having to work hard at delivering task-oriented care, a lack of time to spend talking to patients, and they complained of constantly struggling to complete their work. Other nurses worked unpaid overtime to compensate and stated the situation affected them emotionally and affected their sleep pattern. Within this context, nurses became disillusioned and withdrew professionally. Some nurses resigned from nursing and spoke of 'getting out till things changed'.

The interesting aspect with all of the research reviewed is that the Nursing Process itself is not so much a target of criticism from clinicians, but rather the constraints in the work settings that make it difficult to do it properly in an already busy and challenging day.

SUMMARY AND CONCLUSION

In Australia, the Nursing Process has gone through phases of resistance, acceptance and institutionalization. The present-day status of the Nursing Process is that it is being used in most clinical areas, but it has been mainly reduced to nursing care plan checklists. Initially, the Nursing Process was defined as a problem-solving approach, involving the phases of assessing, planning, implementing and evaluating nursing care, but with the introduction of nursing diagnoses, the Nursing Process is now defined as a five-step approach with the specific inclusion of diagnosis after the assessment phase.

The Nursing Process is highly recommended in nursing practice and education. The Australian Nursing Council Incorporated standards or competencies for a beginning registered nurse require Bachelor of Nursing programmes to teach the Nursing Process and to assess the students' implementation of it in clinical practice. The Nursing Process is also used in the accreditation processes of hospitals and the accepted method of nursing care documentation is based on the Nursing Process. The profession is also constantly adapting the Nursing Process to their particular areas of specialty.

In Australia, the history of the Nursing Process is tied into the movement of nurse education into the tertiary sector. The major impact of the Nursing Process is that it underpins nursing practice within the clinical environment and teaching of nursing to neophyte groups. Problems have been associated with the use of the Nursing Process, but they seem to be more directly reflective of work-setting constraints, rather than shortcomings with the idea of the delivery and documentation of quality nursing care, through a problem-solving approach.

Although relevant national literature and research are scant, it is nevertheless possible to locate a pattern of responses to the use of the Nursing Process, of resistance, acceptance and insitutionalization. There are problems associated with nurses accepting and using the Nursing Process effectively, but at the very least it is enshrined in Australian nursing practice, and at best, nurses may be able to embrace the Nursing Process fully when the contextual constraints are overcome.

REFERENCES

Bowman G S, Thompson D R, Sutton T W 1983 Nurses' attitudes towards the Nursing Process. In: Mostafanejad K 1995 Nursing process: more hype than help? The Australian Nursing Journal 2(9): 36–38

Cook H 1983 Contact nurses and the Nursing Process. The Australian Nurses Journal 13(4): 40–41

Crisp J, Taylor C (eds) Potter and Perry's fundamentals of nursing. Mosby, Sydney

Darbyshire P 2000 The practice and politics of computerised information systems: a focus group study. Nurse Researcher 8(2): 4–17

Doheny M, Cook C, Stopper C 1987 The discipline of nursing: an introduction, 2nd edn. Appleton and Lange, Connecticut

Duffield C, Donoghue J, Pelletier D 1996 Do clinical nurse specialists and nursing unit managers believe that the provision of quality care is important? Journal of Advanced Nursing 24(2): 334–340

Graunke K 1988 Scenario for the future. The Australian Nurses Journal 17(6): 47–49

Lawler J 1991 In search of an Australian identity. In: Gray G, Pratt R (eds) Towards a discipline of nursing. Churchill Livingstone, Melbourne 211–227

Leininger M 1979 Transcultural nursing. Masson Publishing, New York

Lewis T 1988 Leaping the chasm between nursing theory and practice. In: Mostafanejad K (ed.) 1995 Nursing process: more hype than help? The Australian Nursing Journal 2(9): 36–38

Masso M 1990 Nursing process: help or hindrance? Journal of Advanced Nursing 7(3): 12–16

McAllister M 2003 Doing practice differently: solution-focused nursing. Journal of Advanced Nursing 41(6): 528–535

McHugh MK 1987 Has nursing outgrown the Nursing Process? In: Mostafanejad K (ed.) 1995 Nursing process: more hype than help? The Australian Nursing Journal 2(9): 36–38

Mitchell P 1997 An attempt to give nursing home residents a voice in the quality improvement process: the challenge of frailty. Journal of Clinical Nursing 6(6): 453–461

Mostafanejad K 1995 Nursing process: more hype than help? The Australian Nursing Journal 2(9): 36–38

Nicklin P 1984 Innovation without change. In: Mostafanejad K (ed.) 1995 Nursing process: more hype than help? The Australian Nursing Journal 2(9): 36–38

O'Brien B 1988 The nursing process: a mini-course. The Australian Nurses Journal 18(5): 15–16

O'Connell B 1998 The clinical application of the Nursing Process in selected acute care settings: a professional mirage. Australian Journal of Advanced Nursing 15(4): 22–32

O'Connell B 2000 Enabling care: working through obscurity and uncertainty – a basic social process used in selected acute care settings. Australian Journal of Advanced Nursing 17(3): 32–39

Orem D E 1987 Orem's general theory of nursing. In: Parse R R (ed.) Nursing science: major paradigms theories and critiques. W B Saunders, Philadelphia

Orlando I J 1961 The dynamic nurse–patient relationship. Putnam, New York

Owen M, Kelly L 1991 Square pegs in round holes: holism and nursing diagnosis. National Nursing Diagnosis Conference, Gold Coast, Australia

Paech M, Oreo T 1994 The nursing process: a step forward? Contemporary Nurse 3(1): 26–30

Peplau H E 1952 Interpersonal relations in nursing. Putnam, New York

Prideau G 1991 Working with the nursing process: a question of attitude. National Nursing Diagnosis Conference, Gold Coast, Australia

Rogers M E 1970 The theoretical basis of nursing. F A Davis Company, Philadelphia

Roper N, Logan W W, Tierney A J 1980 The elements of nursing. Churchill Livingstone, Edinburgh

Stockdale, M 2000 Is the complexity of care a paradox? Journal of Advanced Nursing 31(5): 1258–1264

Taylor C 2000 Clinical problem-solving in nursing: insights from the literature. Journal of Advanced Nursing 31(4): 842–849

Usher K 1998 Process consent: a model for enhancing informed consent in mental health nursing. Journal of Advanced Nursing 27(4): 692–697

Watson J 1982 Traditional v. tertiary: ideological shifts in nursing education. The Australian Nurses Journal 12(2): 44–46

Yuen F 1986 Broad-based clinical learning experiences: some curricular issues. Journal of Advanced Nursing 11: 339–341

Chapter 9

The Nursing Process in South Africa

Leana R. Uys

CHAPTER CONTENTS

INTRODUCTION

The Nursing Process was defined early in the process of its implementation in South Africa by three local authors. Uys (1977) and Van den Berg (1978) used the definition of the Nursing Process put forward by Yura and Walsh (1967). Van den Berg then identified the following central elements:

1. the client and the client's needs;
2. identification of the needs and help which should be rendered;
3. the intervention by the nurse;
4. the evaluation by the nurse of the results of her intervention;
5. the recording of these steps.

Mashaba, who wrote a few years later, said that 'The Nursing Process is a scientific method of approaching and planning the nursing care of the patient' (Mashaba 1981: 28). The steps she identified were the same as those described by van den Berg. South African authors often credited themselves with adding the fifth step (recording) to the Nursing Process.

Before the Nursing Process was implemented in South Africa, nursing assessment was usually described as the top-to-toe scrutiny of the patient on admission, as well as the taking of vital signs. Diagnosis referred only to a medical diagnosis, and this was what directed nursing care to a large extent. The only plan of nursing care was the nursing 'orders' given by one shift of nurses to the next shift on handover, and this was usually also recorded in the patient's records. Another form of planning was one or more observation sheets that the registered nurse in charge attached to the bed, which detailed for the nurses the frequency and type of observations to be done for that specific patient. Nursing records were done only in the form of a narrative report, three times per day (7 am, midday and 7 pm). Most of this changed during the late 1970s and 1980s with the introduction of the Nursing Process.

HISTORY OF THE NURSING PROCESS IN SOUTH AFRICA

Education

The first instruction on the Nursing Process was offered by the University of the Free State in the middle 1970s. One of the first articles (Uys 1977), was based on a paper read at the provincial forum for nurses from all fields of nursing and midwifery. The presenters from this institution used Mayer's (1972) book as a basic guide, and ran a series of workshops on the topic, which were attended by nurses from all over the country. Their work led to the implementation of the process in the Orange Free State province and it stimulated a range of activities all over the country.

One of the people central to the implementation of the Nursing Process in South Africa is Irene M. Miles. Miles became involved in the implementation of, as she describes it: 'the scientific method of nursing as expressed by the Nursing Process' in 1978. She first assisted with its implementation in Groote Schuur Hospital in Cape Town and was then asked to implement the process in the Livingstone Hospital in Port Elizabeth. According to her account (1984: xv) she 'made a determined effort to co-ordinate the documentation into a system which provided for logical progression, gave structure to the process in a concrete visible way, was open enough to allow for adaptation within the system, yet did not at any time prescribe to the professional nurse what questions to ask, or what specific details to include when care-planning for individuals'. This resulted in the 'Miles Bible', a 5 cm-thick, A4-size file with colour-coded sections addressing the following topics.

1. Condensed guidelines: the basis of nursing.
    1.1. Introduction.
    1.2. Nursing concepts (The process as a tool for education, service and communication).
    1.3. Fundamentals (Systems theory, problem-solving and homeostasis).
2. The system of documentation – this deals with the documents for each step of the process.
3. The Nursing Process system – this deals with each step of the process.
4. Supportive processes – mainly the audit process (1984).

Miles spent the next 5 years running 2-week courses almost continuously over the Cape Province. The strategy was to give a minimum of five such courses during 1 year in the same hospital. In each hospital, a project manager and a committee supported implementation between the visits of the trainer. 'Scientific education for scientific nursing: Nursing Process', the bilingual manual, which was published commercially in 1983, sets out the curriculum for these courses, and gives extensive guidance about the documentation and its use.

Literature

The first mention of the Nursing Process is in two articles that appeared in the December edition of the national nursing journal, *Curationis* – one in English and one in Afrikaans. In the English article, Hammond (1978: 20) describes the Nursing Process as 'a framework through which the nurse can function' to give individualized, total patient care. She further describes the process as using the problem-solving process but being distinct from it. She saw the differences as being in the purpose (new knowledge vs. maximizing the client's wellness) and the methods (problem-solving can be used by an individual, while the Nursing Process demands interpersonal relationships involving at least the nurse and the client). While Hammond endeavours to argue the need for the Nursing Process in terms of marrying the science and art of nursing, van den Berg (1978) makes no effort to give the context of the implementation of the process. She gives a description of the content of the process, which she describes as a way of ensuring that logical and thoroughly thought through care is rendered to the patient. Three years later a similar article was published by Mashaba (1981), in which she also describes the steps of the process. Her focus, however, is the dynamism of the process. She sees it as a tool that facilitates the continuous change and adaptation of the nursing care.

The next two articles appeared in 1983 in the same journal. In both articles, case studies of patients are given, using nursing care plans in the classic format to describe the care. In the first article, Venter and Botha (1983) describe the care of a depressed patient and, in the second, Venter (1982) describes the nursing care of a patient with pre-eclampsia. These authors were all attached to university schools of nursing, so that one can assume that the process was part of the education of students at such institutions by this time. The next one, however, comes from a nurse in practice. She rejects the problem-oriented nursing records on the basis that it fragments the record, making it impossible to get an overall picture of the patient's condition, and also because it is time consuming (Pretorius 1984). This early plea by a practising nurse was not heeded and, in the same year, Venter and du Plooy (1984) published a standard care plan for antenatal patients. They gave credit to a course in the Nursing Process, offered by Miles in the same year.

Research

The first (and only) research article on the Nursing Process appeared in 1987 (Uys 1987). The author surveyed 11 units in six different hospitals, interviewing staff and doing a record review. Most of the nurses interviewed were positive about problem-oriented nursing records, but had long lists of negative comments, mainly centred around time constraints. It was found that history forms were used in only five of the 11 units reviewed, and only in one were such forms completed for all patients. The nursing care plans varied greatly, with most patients being without such plans, or being on standard care plans. Even when they existed, the quality was poor. Common problems included a lack of baseline data to describe the extent of the problem identified, unrealistic outcome statements and 'routine care' given as planned actions.

The author concluded that, while the system created a greater awareness amongst nurses of their own role, and more clarity and system in their thinking, documentation was not greatly improved. Individualization was the exception rather than the rule, and many of the history forms led to question-and-answer interviews not conducive to building a trusting relationship. Since the average registered nurse to patient ratio was 1 : 17.5, she also concluded that an individualized, written, nursing care plan was not a realistic expectation. She recommended that a problem list be used and only highly individualistic nursing interventions be noted. She also recommended the discontinuation of writing objectives and for standard care plans to be available as a reference only (Uys 1987: 30).

In a re-examination of the Nursing Process in 1990, du Toit and Dewar identified four principles of the Nursing Process: individualized holistic care; involving the patient and significant others in the planning of care; a concise and efficient documentation system; and fostering teamwork. They then made recommendations with regard to all steps of the Nursing Process to make it more efficient and effective without losing these important elements.

Although the Nursing Process is often linked to the professionalization of nursing, when Thompson wrote in 1983 about the goal of nursing to achieve professional status, she did not refer to the Nursing Process anywhere in the article. Similarly, when Kotze et al tried to conceptualize the academic discipline of nursing science in 1989, they did not refer to this concept at all.

CURRENT UTILIZATION

Textbooks

Over the last three decades, a range of basic nursing and midwifery textbooks were published in South Africa. Most of the clinical textbooks came from the University of the Free State, and followed their perspective of the Nursing Process. Most textbooks have a chapter about the Nursing Process, and the nursing care plan is often used to describe the nursing care to be given to patients with a specific problem or illness (Uys and Mulder 1985, Viljoen and Uys 1987, Viljoen and Uys 1989, Uys 1992). In 1988, this university also published a self-study guide on the Nursing Process, which systematically took the student through the four steps (Joubert 1988). In the same year, Viljoen published a book on nursing assessment, which included a total physical assessment. This book is still in use.

The regulatory body

The South African Nursing Council is the statutory body that regulates the professions of nursing and midwifery in South Africa. It was established through the Nursing Act, and it has the functions of setting educational standards, accrediting educational schools and programmes, licensing nurses and midwives annually, and maintaining professional discipline.

In the instruments the South African Nursing Council uses for the review of nursing schools, the Nursing Process is prominent in the section that is used to review the clinical facilities in which students are placed for experiential learning. Here, the following items appear:

A comprehensive and accurate nursing assessment of individuals and groups in a variety of settings is carried out by

- The use of a systematic approach in the process of assessment
- Analysis of data and identification of findings.

Opportunities are available and accompaniment is provided for students to:

- Formulate a plan of care in consultation with individuals and groups.
- Implement planned care.
- Evaluate progress toward expected outcomes.
- Review plans in accordance with data evaluated.

(South African Nursing Council 1999: 23–24)

In practice

Rather than try to do an overview of how the Nursing Process is used currently in nursing practice all over the country, I decided to look at the two hospitals most closely associated with its initial implementation in the country. Miles implemented the process in Livingstone Hospital in Port Elizabeth, and in Bloemfontein it was implemented in the Universitas Hospital, which was closely associated with the Free State University.

Livingstone Hospital

In this hospital, the system was implemented in the paediatric medical units in 1978, and involved discontinuing the old Cardex system, and implementation of the total system of ten forms. Full-time coordinators, weekly training, monthly meetings and a three-monthly audit supported implementation. The Nursing Process was implemented in the whole hospital, except for the obstetric units and operating theatres, by the end of 1979. At this stage (the 1980s), the hospital was very satisfied with aspects of the system. It was a much more comprehensive patient record, incorporated a holistic approach to the patient, and was systematic. The process stimulated nurses to think about what they did and increased the input of nurses in multidisciplinary discussions about patients. There was an increase in the teaching and learning on the units: nurses referred to textbooks when they were confronted with aspects they did not understand, and consulted and taught one another. Nurses also became more accountable for the care decisions they made, and discharge planning was actively incorporated into nursing care via the Nursing Process. One of the triumphs of the Nursing Process was when the hospital and a doctor were involved in a negligence suit, and the meticulous record-keeping by the nurses saved the institution from a massive claim.

Not everything, however, was going smoothly. Some nurses found it a very difficult process to master. They had difficulty formulating problems effectively, to the extent that, on many patient records, it was difficult to identify what the problem(s) were. Care prescriptions were also activated indiscriminately on checklists and nurses found it difficult to adhere to timelines stipulated on care plans. Nurses found the records too detailed and comprehensive, and had no time to complete them all. Instead of leading to comprehensive nursing care, the process led to a focus on pieces of paper, rather than on the individuals being cared for. Owing to the low nurse–patient ratios, primary allocation was done only during the morning shift and task allocation during the rest of the day. Looking back, the nurse managers feel that many of the problems might have been caused by the top-down process of implementation, and the highly critical approach to staff of the project manager (not Ms Miles) from the Head Office.

In the late 1980s, the first review of the system was done. Half of the documents were eliminated to make the system more user-friendly, and zone supervisors took over from full-time coordinators. A simple guide to the use of the system was written to replace the Miles Bible.

In 1994, a second revision was begun, which was only concluded in 1999. By this time, much had changed in the hospital. In the early 1990s, nursing posts were frozen in an effort to decrease government spending and, over the next few years, almost 50% of nursing positions were lost. It was essential to find new ways of doing things. This review involved all role players and involved trying to create a uniform document across all government hospitals. Nurses were very actively involved, and created a system they felt they could manage and which did the job. Currently, the nursing documentation consists of a one-page nursing assessment form, a very brief nursing care plan, a progress report form and a discharge planning form. Most nurses can manage the simplified system and all categories of nurses take part in all steps of the process.

It is still a challenge to maintain an adequate nursing record. At night, the nurse–patient ratio is 2:45, while in paediatric units it is 3:30, and in maternity units 2:60. High acuity levels of patients and high turnover does not make things easier. Nursing audits indicate that, for very ill patients, the recording is done at a very high level (80–90%) but, for the less seriously ill patients, the audit shows recording levels of as low as 17%. Nurses find themselves having to prioritize, and they place direct care first, then recording of care.

Nurses in this hospital generally believe that the Nursing Process produces a high standard of nursing records. In effect, nurses have become the documentors of patient care, not just nursing care.

Universitas Hospital

When the system was implemented 20 years ago, it consisted of a brief nursing assessment form, and depended strongly on Standard Care Plans, with nurses only planning for 'unusual problems', as defined by Mayers (1972). This approach was followed for the first ten years but, in 1991–1992, a major renewal was done based on a masters research study and the perception that nurses were not seeing individuals, but only 'cases'. This was a provincewide initiative that was coordinated by a Documentation Committee at the provincial head office. It was decided to move to individual care plans with standard care plans being used only for reference purposes. They also decided to use Roper's activities of living as a basis for assessment and planning, and NANDA (North American Nursing Diagnosis Association) as the basis for nursing diagnoses. At this time, a quality assurance unit was also established in the hospital.

The current documentation system consists of the following four forms.

- A one-page nursing history form, which is based on Roper's model, and which consists of ticking off normal findings, and writing out only those that need attention.
- A one-page care plan form, which has space for a list of problems and nursing actions according to activities of living. It again makes provision for ticking off items that regularly appear, such as observations to be done, and only demands the writing of other actions.

- A progress-report form, where the nurse reports progress in terms of the problems and care plan.
- A one-page discharge assessment sheet.

The policy is that only registered nurses do nursing assessment and planning, and complete the discharge sheet. Other categories of nurses (enrolled nurses and nursing auxiliaries) may write the progress reports. The management of this hospital have recently realized that other categories of nurses often do assessment on admission, and are now starting to train them as well.

The hospital is associated with two nursing schools, a college and a university. While both currently base their teaching on the system used by the hospital, the University is exploring a different approach from Roper's, and may change in future.

One nurse working in the Staff Development unit currently supports the system and she works closely with the audit unit. Every registered nurse appointed at the hospital attends a 2-day orientation to the system of documentation. Once a month, a further 2-day course is offered, which is open to all registered nurses.

The audit unit reviews 10% of the total patients discharged from a unit every month. Their audit tool is one developed and tested by Uys and Booyens in 1989. If the unit identifies problems, a report is sent to the Staff Development Coordinator, who investigates and takes appropriate action.

The problems, as defined by the Staff Development manager and the Audit unit manager, are as follows.

- The nursing care plan is done initially, but is never updated. The audit managers said: 'When you audit the document, you see three different patients; the one described in the admission form, the one written about in the progress notes and the one described in the discharge form, with no connection among the three'. The progress report is not written in terms of the problems identified on the Nursing Care Plan, which are often never referred to again. The detail of aspects covered in the discharge form is often not found on the progress report. This leads to a wide variation of the quality of documentation between the different stages. In one month, for instance, the average audit percentage for the assessment at admission for seven units was 85%, and for the nursing care plan 82%, but only 56% for the progress report.
- Nurses are resistant to the documentation which is required. They see it as 'paperwork', which is not important. They also think that the more you write the more you can be criticized, even legally. Nurses are criticized for their care based on their own assessment data. There is a perception that the assessment data leave the nurse open to criticism, especially in a situation where a shortage of staff makes it impossible to document care comprehensively.
- Students and registered nurses find the issue of making a nursing diagnosis difficult. Even fourth year students cannot come to a well-formulated nursing diagnosis, and they find this an abstract process, rather than a logical, empirical one.

After some prompting, two managers agreed that the process has improved the discharge planning, and that it has given a guideline that structures nursing. If a record audit is used, as in their case, the process makes negligence visible and allows it to be addressed. This they believe was not possible before the process-linked documentation was implemented. They do not really think that the assessment assists nurses in knowing their patients better, since it is done by one person, and not referred to by others.

CONCLUSION

It does not seem reasonable to expect the Nursing Process to 'go away'. It seems to be firmly entrenched in nursing textbooks and in the regulatory framework of the country. Having made nurses conscious of the need for assessment and a nursing diagnosis, it has perhaps made its major contribution in the conceptualization of nursing. It also seems as though it has changed certain aspects of the functioning of nurses permanently, especially the idea of a thorough nursing assessment, a nursing diagnosis and discharge planning.

The review of the Nursing Process in South Africa raises a few questions. Firstly, one has to accept that, in a middle-income country, only the minimum of nurses is often available to provide care. Does the Nursing Process documentation make such a difference to quality of care that it should be implemented in the face of staff shortages? If one has to choose between direct care and documentation, is this format the most efficient? A second question is whether the continued frustration of nurses about their inability to get an efficient Nursing Process implemented is not adding to the stress of nurses, and causing unnecessary friction between managers and clinicians? Is the process really worth the resources spent on it? Is it not possible to make some adjustments to the implementation of the process that will make it more realistic and bring reality closer to theory?

REFERENCES

Du Toit R, Dewar S 1990 Re-examining the Nursing Process: part one. Nursing RSA Verpleging 5(9): 7–11

Du Toit R, Dewar S 1990 Re-examining the Nursing Process: part two Patient assessment – the basis of care. Nursing RSA Verpleging 5(9): 26–27

Hammond M 1978 The Nursing Process. Curationis 1(3): 19–23

Joubert A (ed) 1988 The Nursing Process. A self study guide. PJ de Villiers, Bloemfontein

Kotze W J, Searle C, Uys L R 1989 A conceptual model of the academic discipline nursing science. Curationis 12(1+2): 1–4

Mashaba T G 1981 The dynamics of the Nursing Process. Curationis 4(1): 28–32

Mayers M G 1972 A systematic approach to the nursing care plan. Appleton-Century Crofts, New York

Miles I M 1984 Scientific education for scientific nursing: Nursing Process. Juta, Cape Town

Pretorius E 1984 Die pasientvorderingsverslag as kommunikasiemiddel. Curationis 7(1): 9–12

South African Nursing Council 1999 Accreditation of nursing education institutions and programmes. South African Nursing Council, Pretoria

Thompson R A E 1983 Achieving professionalism. Curationis 6(3): 10–13

Uys L R 1977 Die verpleegproses en die verpleegsorgplan. South African Journal of Nursing XLIV (7): 11–14

Uys L R 1987 The implementation of problem-oriented nursing records in selected general hospitals in Natal. Curationis 10(4): 28–31

Uys L R (ed.) 1992 Psychiatric nursing. A South African perspective. Juta, Kenwyn

Uys L R, Booyens S W 1989 Standards for nursing documentation in general hospitals in South Africa. Curationis 12(1&2): 29–31

Uys L R, Mulder M (eds) 1985 Nursing: humane, scientific health care. HAUM, Pretoria

Van den Berg R H 1978 Die verpleegproses. Curationis 1(3): 41–78

Venter I, Botha S E 1983 Mnr Smit leer ons iets. Curationis 6(2): 32–34

Venter S 1982 Verpleegsorgplan vir'n pasient met pre-eklampsie. Curationis 6(2): 40–44

Venter S, du Plooy P 1984 Standaard verpleegvoorskrifte vir voorgeboorte kliente. Curationis 7(4): 41–53

Viljoen M J 1988 Nursing assessment: history-taking and the physical examination. HAUM, Pretoria

Viljoen M J, Uys L R (eds) 1987 General nursing: medical-surgical textbook. Part one. HAUM, Pretoria

Viljoen M J, Uys L R (eds) 1989 General nursing: medical-surgical textbook. Part two. HAUM, Pretoria

Yura H, Walsh M B 1967 The Nursing Process. Appleton-Century-Crofts, Washington DC

Chapter 10

The Nursing Process in the Caribbean

Hermi Hewitt

INTRODUCTION

Because of their colonial and neocolonial past, Caribbean countries have been greatly influenced by the concepts, theories and principles that emanate from the systems of colonial powers. Nursing in Caribbean countries consequently had its education and practice shaped by outside forces. In the 19th and early 20th centuries, the influence for nursing education and practice came from Great Britain. Since the latter part of the 20th century, the major sources of influence for nursing education and practice have been the USA and, to a lesser extent, Canada. The most common avenue was through nurses who received their education and experiences in Canada and the USA, and subsequently diffused these into the Caribbean.

The regional institution that has had the greatest impact in introducing new nursing knowledge in the English-speaking Caribbean, is the Department of Advanced Nursing Education (DANE), formerly the Advanced Nursing Unit (ANEU), the University of the West Indies (UWI), Mona Campus, Jamaica. The ANEU was established at the UWI in 1966 to prepare nursing educators and nursing administrators to lead nursing education and management in the Caribbean. Prior to DANE's existence, small numbers of nurses were periodically sent to Britain to be educated as Sister Tutors or Nursing Administrators. To date, DANE/UWI remains the focal education institution for developing nursing leadership in the Caribbean.

THE INTRODUCTION OF THE NURSING PROCESS

Between 1966 and 1971, Dr Rae Chittick, a Canadian nurse, and Miss Bridgette Haugland, a British nurse, were the main leaders who influenced the education of DANE's students. In 1971, Dr Mary Jane Seivwright, a Jamaican nurse who received her university education at Teachers College, Columbia University, USA, took up the directorship of DANE. Ms Syringa Marshall-Burnett, another Jamaican nurse who received her undergraduate and graduate education at the University of Toronto and New York University, respectively, joined her shortly after. These nurses transformed the curriculum by introducing their learning into the programmes offered at the DANE/UWI. Consequently, the books and materials that they had been exposed to, and the expertise and experiences they had gained overseas, formed the basis of their terms of reference in educating Caribbean nurses. An example of their influence is that shortly after Yura and Walsh published their book, *The Nursing Process: assessing, planning, implementing, evaluating,* (1973), it became a focal point for discussion among students pursuing nursing education and nursing administration at the DANE/UWI.

By 1978, one of the prescribed texts for nursing education and nursing administration students at the DANE/UWI was *The Nursing Process: a scientific approach to nursing care* by Marriner, published in 1975. The author made the point that 'the nursing process is the application of scientific problem solving to nursing care, described the classification of the steps as assessment, planning, implementation and evaluation' (Marriner 1975: 1). The author also emphasized that the Nursing Process is used to solve nursing problems and drew on the work of other professional colleagues to explain the problem-solving process and the steps of the Nursing Process. While it was obvious to nurses that nursing is an art, there was always controversy about its being a science. Marriner's postulate provided an engaging point for analysis of nursing as a science. The Nursing Process, therefore, provided the framework to justify the scientific aspect of nursing because the concept was introduced as the scientific approach to nursing care.

Another compelling development that furthered the knowledge of Caribbean nurses regarding the Nursing Process was the introduction of the post-registered nurse Bachelor of Science Nursing (BScN) degree at DANE in 1983. It was in this programme that nursing theory was introduced as a module of the nursing curriculum. The instructor for this module was Grant, an American nurse recruited for this programme. The prescribed textbook was *Nursing Theories: the base for professional nursing practice*, compiled by the Nursing Theories Conference Group and chaired by George (1980). This book contained an overview of the Nursing Process and described the extended nursing process, from four to five steps. It also provided a description of each nursing theory and the application of the Nursing Process from each theorist's perspective. This exposed nurses to several theorists, provided wider perspectives and a greater number of frameworks from which to apply nursing practice. It also allowed more scope for the selection of preferences and the opportunity for critical analysis. It was also at this time that controversy arose regarding the added phase of the Nursing Process, which was the nursing diagnosis. The language of the Nursing Process and the nursing theories became a challenge, but a good avenue for discussion and assimilation.

The proliferation of literature about the Nursing Process between 1980 and 1990 exposed more nurses to a variety of views about the Nursing Process, including many contending views, which generated much discussion among nurses at DANE. An area of discontent was the change from four to five phases in the Nursing Process. It also became evident that there were variations of interpretations of nursing diagnoses. A number of nurses had difficulty in accepting the language used in the nursing diagnosis phase. The assessment met no resistance, as nurses were accustomed to collecting objective and subjective data. Further, the assessment phase assisted nurses to be more methodical in what they formerly did. It guided nurses to a greater clarity in determining what data to collect and the logical sequence for collecting complete data to improve the quality of patient care. It also supplied the evidence that was necessary for comprehensive nursing care.

The planning, implementation and evaluation phases were quickly embraced, as these were familiar activities that nurses were accustomed to do. When the four-phased Nursing Process was initiated, the problem identification or nursing diagnosis was subsumed within the planning phase, making this obscure and less controversial. When these were separated, giving Nursing Diagnosis its own identity, responses were mixed. Apart from introducing new nomenclature for nurses, the proposed list of diagnoses provided by the North American Nursing Diagnosis Association (NANDA) was unfamiliar. Nurses felt that the diagnosis had too many parts, that is, a problem plus aetiology and symptoms. Another comment was that the language is unwieldy, for example, 'alteration' and 'impaired' were considered unfamiliar ways of expressing patients' states.

The knowledge and practice application that nurses were taught at DANE were disseminated into their practices throughout the Caribbean. Knowledge about the Nursing Process produced a ripple effect in nurses throughout the region. This was evident when the nursing curricula of the 13 Caribbean Community (CARICOM) countries were revised between 1978 and 1986. Each curriculum representative from the CARICOM countries was a DANE graduate. Hence the Nursing Process was the modality chosen for nursing care in the curricula. The curriculum change was led by Dr Una Reid, Pan American Health Organization/World Health Organization Nurse Advisor, a graduate of the University of Alberta, Canada, and Teachers College, Columbia University, USA. The new curriculum created a paradigm shift in nursing education and practice in the Caribbean, reflecting that which pertained in North America.

It can be deduced that the Nursing Process was introduced at an opportune time when nurses sought a frame of reference on which to base their scope of practice. Therefore, nurses welcomed the concept of the Nursing Process, as it assisted them to give meaning to their profession, distinguish their practice and provided an explicit framework that confirmed their identity as practitioners within the health care delivery system. Another important factor for Caribbean nurses enthusiastically embracing the introduction of the Nursing Process was that it provided a focal point around which nurses for the first time could claim a common nursing vocabulary. Nurses also identified with the Nursing Process, as it provided order, form and content to delineate their work.

THE CURRENT SITUATION

The Nursing Process has been implemented in practice for many years and it is timely to explore the views of nurses regarding its applicability to practice. A small survey was done among Jamaican nurses to elicit their views regarding the use of the Nursing Process in their practice.

Methodology

To attain a perspective of the extent to which the Nursing Process is diffused into nurses' practice in Jamaica, a cross-section of nurses, representing nursing administration, nursing education, public health nursing, and midwifery in both primary and secondary health care settings were asked to complete a questionnaire. These represented practising nurses in the South East Health Region Authority (SEHRA) of Jamaica who were attending a field agency meeting. SEHRA serves a population of 1214648 of the 2.5 million population (Ministry of Health 2001).

A ten-item questionnaire developed specifically for the survey sought to elicit data about the Nursing Process. The items were examined for face and content validity by circulating the items to the scrutiny of persons considered experts who taught the Nursing Process and had experience in applying the Nursing Process in their practice. Based on these persons' comments, the items were refined to reflect suggestions prior to administering the questionnaire to participants.

The questionnaire was self-administered with the investigator present to clarify points and answer any questions that the respondents had. The questionnaire addressed the following areas: how nurses knew about the Nursing Process; whether or not they were currently using the Nursing Process in their practice; how easy it was; what they liked most and least about each phase of the Nursing Process; if, in its present form, the Nursing Process was useful for nursing education, clinical nursing practice, nursing management and what changes they would make to the Nursing Process to make it more useful for their particular area of practice.

Additional nurses who were known by the investigator to have views on the Nursing Process were asked through telephone conversations, e-mails and informal conversations to indicate their perspective of nursing with specific reference to their practice. Pertinent Caribbean documents that nurses use to guide their practice were also reviewed for evidence of the Nursing Process. Both oral and written responses from respondents and documented evidence form the basis for discussion in this paper.

Because of time limits, financial constraints and the geographic spread of the Caribbean, only nurses from Jamaica could be included in the survey. It was also a convenient sample and, therefore, cannot be generalized. The sample did, however, represent views from all the practice areas of nursing and, therefore, provides some baseline for further scientific investigation.

The responses and discussion are categorized according to definitions, enforcement of the Nursing Process, the fields in nursing in which the Nursing Process is used and problems related to implementation of the process. Many nurses indicated that the systematic and logical flow of the process provided a guiding framework for nursing practice and a common vocabulary with which nurses could identify and of which they could claim ownership.

Definitions

The most prevailing definitions are that the Nursing Process is a systematic, logically structured, problem-solving method for nurses, a tool that helps to plan care: 'it is a tool that is effective and easy to use'; and 'it assists the nurse to organize the patient position on the health illness continuum, and to make nursing intervention'. Several nurses indicated that it is the knowledge base for all nurses and 'allows for standardization of care'. Most nurses also indicate that it is a dynamic process and 'a good nursing management tool'.

Enforcement of the Nursing Process

The Nursing Council of Jamaica (NCJ), a statutory organization with legal jurisdiction for nurses' examination, registration, relicensure and practice, approves the curriculum for nurses' education and training. Consequently, the NCJ approves the Nursing Process as the modality for teaching and delivering nursing care in Jamaica. Since 1993, nurses in CARICOM take the same Regional Examination for Nurse Registration (RENR) to be qualified as registered nurses. The blueprint guiding the RENR, which formed the organizing framework for the nurses' curriculum, adopted the Nursing Process as its organizing framework for nursing care delivery (CARICOM Secretariat 1983). The Nursing Process remains the critical continuous element in the RENR. Schools of nursing teach and implement the Nursing Process. In every student–patient encounter, a nursing care plan has to be developed. Internal examinations for nurse registration require students to answer items on the Nursing Process inclusive of developing nursing care plans.

The Caribbean Standards of Nursing Care stipulates in one of its philosophical statements that 'Client care is individualized through the Nursing Process' (PAHO/WHO 1983: 4). There is a National Standards Committee that recommends policy for nursing in Jamaica. The Committee uses the Nursing Process framework in developing instruments for clinical nursing practice, which are approved at the Ministry of Health level.

Despite the fact that implementation workshops are conducted, these tools are not always consistently used in all clinical settings. Some of the constraints to use in the clinical area related to material resources. Although Government, through the Ministry of Health, approves the recommendations of the National Standards Committee, there is insufficient paper to meet the documentation needs consistently.

The fields of nursing in which the Nursing Process is used

In Jamaica, the Nursing Process is mainly used in the fields of education, administration, hospital clinical service and community health, although it is not used to the same extent in all areas. The Nursing Process is fully integrated in the education of basic nursing students who are required to have a thorough understanding of the Nursing Process prior to being certified competent to take the RENR. The clinical objectives for these students reflect the Nursing Process.

Although registered nurses express the importance of the Nursing Process in clinical practice, there is very little evidence in its use in nurses' documentation. One of the uses stated was that it allows the nurse to re-evaluate plans of action so that 'the client will get the best care possible'. The assessment phase of the Nursing Process had the greatest level of support. Most clinicians indicate that the assessment phase helps them:

- 'to plan and identify priorities';
- 'allows for the development of good interpersonal relations with clients and collecting data on which other phases depend';
- 'helps you to have a thorough knowledge of the problem to be addressed';
- 'ensures that all aspects of the client are addressed';
- 'provides information and resources about the individual/family community that are necessary to solve the affecting problem';
- 'this is the initial phase and other components are planned from this phase';

- 'it is the foundation of the Nursing Process';
- 'in making good observations the nurse will be able to make rational and wise nursing interventions';
- 'at this phase one learns about the patient social, spiritual background';
- 'one also learns the family history and physical status of ill patients';
- 'this is the base on which to know what you are dealing with and then to plan care';
- 'you can only evaluate if you know where you started';
- 'necessary for continuity of care'.

Nursing managers indicate that the Nursing Process is a valuable tool for organizing nursing care. Some managers use the Nursing Process as the guiding framework for developing job descriptions.

Problems related to the Nursing Process

Nursing diagnosis presented the most difficulty among nurses and also in the medical fraternity. Initially, the assessment phase ended with a list of client/patient problem(s). Both nurses and physicians accepted this without resistance. When the nursing diagnosis phase was introduced, some nurses and physicians were incensed as they were socialized into the belief that the word 'diagnosis' was a sacred word only to be used by the medical profession. Consequently, both sets of health practitioners saw it as a desecration of a sacred right of physicians. A massive education campaign to get nurses to accept the word 'diagnosis' as a standard English word with no special conferred right of exclusive use by individuals or groups greatly reduced the resistance of nurses' use. The introduction of the five-step process into the curriculum allowed new nurses to be more accepting of the process. With time, most nurses have accepted the formulation of the nursing diagnosis as a necessary part of the Nursing Process.

Attitude

The nursing diagnosis remains the phase that is least liked by nurses. Older nurses use the Nursing Process less than newer nurses. The problem that still remains is the language used in the nursing diagnosis phase. Both nursing students and nurses feel the wording is tedious, torturous and does not represent their normal vocabulary. Nurses indicate that the current jargon expressed as nursing diagnoses are peculiar to North Americans, who need to use them because of legal implications. Words such as 'alteration' and 'deficit' are not easily embraced.

Some of the comments received from respondents are: 'I find it difficult to formulate'; 'it is too round about'; 'terminology not easily understood for replication'; 'the nursing diagnosis area needs to be taught in such a way that it is understood and can be easily applied'; and 'too many words'. Some respondents expressed that developing the plan was '. . . time-consuming in present practice, hence nurses see it as an interference in patient care, rather than a useful tool in affecting quality care'.

CONCLUSION

The Nursing Process is used in the Caribbean and has been an integral part of nursing education and training since the early 1970s. The major obstacle preventing full implementation of the Nursing Process is that nurses are uncomfortable with the language used in the nursing diagnosis phase. It is, therefore, incumbent on nursing leaders of the Caribbean to formulate diagnoses that are culturally specific for the region.

REFERENCES

CARICOM Secretariat 1983 Blueprint: regional examination for nurse registration CARICOM Member Countries 1983. CARICOM Secretariat, Georgetown, Guyana

George J (ed.) 1980 Nursing theories: the base for professional nursing practice. Prentice-Hall, Englewood Cliffs, NJ

Marriner A 1975 The nursing process: a scientific approach to nursing care. Mosby, St Louis

Ministry of Health 2001 Ministry of Health: strategic plan 2001–2005. MOH, Kingston

PAHO/WHO 1983 Report: Caribbean standards of nursing care for Ministries of Health Commonwealth Caribbean. CARICOM Secretariat, Georgetown, Guyana

Yura H, Walsh M 1973 The nursing process: assessing, planning, implementing, evaluating. Appleton-Century-Crofts, New York

Chapter 11

The Nursing Process in the Czech Republic

Alena Mellanová

CHAPTER CONTENTS

INTRODUCTION

Nursing is viewed by the Czech government as playing an indispensable role in health care (Ministry of Health 1998). Both in the community and in hospital care, nursing has shaped its own scope of practice in which the nurse acts more or less independently. The characteristic features of nursing include individualized care based on identifying nursing needs and systematically satisfying the nursing needs of the individual/family/group, the independent work of the nurse in both hospital care and nursing community services rendered at the client's home, health promotion and health education.

Nursing is defined as a system of specific caring activities concerning the individual, families or groups, which assist them to take care of their health and well-being (Ministry of Health 1998). Generally, nursing aims include the maintenance and promotion of health, the restoration of health and progressive development of self-sufficiency, alleviation of the suffering of the dying, and ensuring peaceful dying and death. Nursing significantly participates in prevention, diagnostics, therapy and rehabilitation. The nurse assists the individual and groups to cater for their own basic physiological, psychosocial and spiritual needs. The nurse leads the patient towards self-care and educates the people close to the patient in the support of the patient. For the patients who cannot or will not take care of themselves and/or those who do not know how to do so, the nurse renders professional nursing care.

The main objectives of nursing include the search for suitable methods to satisfy, in a systematic and all-round fashion, the needs of the person in terms of maintaining his or her health as well as those needs arising from a changed health status (Ministry of Health 1998). In their efforts to accomplish these objectives, nurses work closely with physicians and other health professionals, such as physiotherapists and occupational therapists, social workers, dietary nurses and others.

The history of nursing, nursing education and practice in the Czech Republic is embedded in the political history of this former Soviet satellite. The country was part of the former Czechoslovakia from just after World War I, and survived in that form for 75 years. After World War II, it became a Soviet satellite, until a series of internal events led to the resignation of the communist government in December 1989. A coalition government took over in the same month, and the process of democratization began. This led to the establishment of the Czech Republic on the 1 January 1993.

HISTORY OF NURSING EDUCATION PRIOR TO 1990

Nursing was one of the first professions in Czechoslovakia that systematically educated its members (since 1916), and whose education was inspected and regulated by the state. Nursing education was, in the beginning, fully comparable with nursing education internationally. It was a prestigious position to be a certified nurse in Czechoslovakia between the two wars. Nurses from that era significantly influenced the progress of Czech nursing in both hospitals and the community, since the system of community care was created by the nurses.

The Public Nursing School, with a programme lasting 2 years, was opened in Prague during the World War I in 1916. This school continued its activities after the war and it served as a model school for all subsequent nursing schools (some of the schools were affiliated to convents, some were not). The first school had a high professional standard. Three experienced American nurses were invited to create the practical and theoretical curriculum.

This positive development was disrupted by World War II but was not derailed. The demand for qualified nursing staff increased during and after the war. The number of public nursing schools grew. By 1947, there were 26 nursing schools in Czechoslovakia.

In 1946, a Higher Nursing School was opened in Prague. It offered specialization in education for nurses who wanted to become teachers at the nursing schools, or specialization in management for nursing managers. This school was very progressive, considering the time when it was opened.

The successful development of Czech nursing education was fundamentally changed by the communist takeover in 1948. Nursing schools were transformed into nursing high (secondary) schools following the Soviet model. In these schools, the following was typical.

- Both general and professional subjects were studied, which allowed coverage of only 50% of the information in each area.
- The students were young and immature, since they were 14–15 years old when starting the programme and 18–19 years old when qualified as nurses.
- There was a focus on medical knowledge, and technical and instrumental skills at the expense of psychosocial content and cognitive skills.
- The education was very expensive because many students realized during the programme that they did not want to work as nurses, and thus never entered the workforce.
- The pedagogical methods corresponded with the young age of the students.

The history of nursing education in the country can be illustrated further by looking at the history of the Institute of Nursing Theory and Practice, Charles University, Prague (hereafter referred to as 'the Institute'). The Institute, established 44 years ago, is the oldest Department of Nursing at a University in the Czech Republic. The department started its activity in the academic year 1959/1960, when the subject of 'patient care' was added to the curriculum of the medical program. The lesson plans were created by the staff of the Institute, which had just been founded. The main goal of this subject was to present nursing to the medical students as a substantial part of clinical medicine and to demonstrate its scientific base. Charles University was, without a doubt, the world's pioneer in teaching nursing skills to medical students.

At the same time, the master's program for nursing teachers began, at the request of two ministries, the Ministry of Health and Ministry of Education. It was a double-major programme in psychology and nursing care. It was offered in the School of Philosophy at Charles University, because only physicians could be educated at medical schools at that time, but the Medical School had to ensure the quality of the specific subjects.

Between the years 1960 and 1980, the programme was offered only part time, but in 1981 it became possible to study in a full-time programme. A total of 620 students graduated from the master's program during its existence. They mostly worked in teaching positions at nursing schools. These nursing teachers had an equivalent level of university education as the other teachers at the nursing schools (i.e. teachers of general subjects and physicians) and a significant number of the graduates also worked as nursing managers.

This programme in nursing care and psychology helped to improve Czech nursing education and nursing practice in general, and made Czechoslovakia the second European country (after Scotland) to offer nurses and midwives a university education.

RECENT HISTORY OF NURSING EDUCATION

The HOPE (Health Opportunity for People Everywhere) Project experts from the USA arrived in the Czech and Slovak Federal Republic in autumn 1990 to survey the Czech and Slovak health care system after the political changes of 1990. Their task was to find out if the new country was ready to embark on modernizing the health care system. In May 1991, an international conference for nursing education was organized in Bratislava by the HOPE Project experts. All of the former USSR satellites sent representatives to participate in work groups to identify the most suitable forms of nursing education required. These groups consequently agreed on priorities and the ways in which they should be implemented.

The Czech representatives asked the HOPE Project to help launch a bachelor's programme in nursing at Charles University. The small Nursing Care Unit at this university worked with the experts to engineer two important changes:

- the transfer of the programme from the School of Philosophy to the School of Medicine
- the introduction of a new bachelor's degree in nursing care.

In 1991, an independent Institute of Nursing Theory and Practice was established, thus replacing the small and previously dependent Nursing Care Unit.

The employees of the Institute cooperated closely and intensively with the HOPE Project experts and designed a curriculum for the bachelor's programme. The outcomes, lesson plans and the number of hours allocated to each subject in the programme were comparable with the directives of the European Union (EU) and the World Health Organisation (WHO). At the same time, seven new textbooks for the bachelor's programme were prepared. In autumn 1991, a programme proposal was submitted to the Dean's Advisory Board, which approved it on 25 November 1991. The first full-time course started in the school year 1992–1993. The period before the programme proposal was accepted by the authorities was very difficult and, for that reason, the approval of the bachelor's programme was considered a major achievement. The oldest medical school in middle Europe, which for hundreds of years had educated only future physicians, opened its doors to nurses and to other health professionals. In the next couple of years, five medical schools and two schools of social studies introduced bachelor's programmes in nursing.

The first entrance examinations were held on 13 July 1992 and 120 potential students applied to the programme. In the next year, there were 274 applicants. Critics of the programme, who had been afraid of insufficient demand were proved wrong. The part-time programme was launched in 1993, which provided the opportunity to study for nurses who did not want to or could not leave their jobs. It is clear now that, even with all of the difficulties, the decision to insist on the opening of the bachelor's programme for nurses was correct because it has certainly improved the quality of nursing performed by the few hundreds of nurses who have already graduated. So far, there have been 350 graduates from the First Medical School of Charles University, with about 150 students currently studying there.

Currently, all of the European countries, including the countries of the former Soviet block that are preparing to join the EU, subscribe to the EU and WHO recommendations with regard to nursing education. Reforms of the educational system are being developed and implemented, with one primary goal – to improve the quality of nursing care. From 2004, the secondary school training of nurses will be discontinued in the Czech Republic, and the only possible avenues to a nursing qualification will be:

- a higher nursing schools (college) programme lasting 3 years; or
- a bachelor's programme in nursing at six different schools of medicine, two social studies schools, and at a few independent colleges (which are not a part of a university).

Higher nursing schools have existed in the Czech Republic since 1996. Their programme is designed for high-school graduates and it qualifies them in a chosen area of nursing (general nursing, paediatric nursing, mental health nursing, etc). The graduates earn the title 'certified specialist', or specifically, 'certified nurse', 'certified paediatric nurse', 'certified mental health nurse', 'certified midwife', etc. Specializations, such as 'intensive care nurse', are sometimes offered at higher nursing schools but they are not compatible with EU directives.

As the educational programmes in nursing are being unified, the free movement of the nurses to seek work opportunities in other countries is becoming easier. The Czech Republic is, however, some way behind most of its European counterparts, as it is one of the last countries still to educate nurses at nursing high schools. Also, despite the practical advances in nursing education, the Czech Republic still lacks a guiding concept at political level for governing the necessary changes.

THE NURSING PROCESS IN THE CZECH REPUBLIC

In order to describe the current thinking about the Nursing Process in the Czech Republic, information was gathered from the academic staff of the

Institute of Nursing Theory and Practice at the Charles University. This group has a thorough insight into the Czech nursing situation, owing to its close contacts with both former and current students (part-time and full-time students) of the bachelor programme in nursing, who live and work throughout the country and in different nursing positions. The nurse teachers see the Nursing Process as a special way that the nurse thinks and works, which leads to individualized care of a client, or a methodical procedure that ensures that the client's needs are assessed and met.

Introduction

In the early 1980s, our Institute started to cooperate with the WHO Nursing Department in Copenhagen. We participated in a research project concerning the needs of 112 hospitalized people and satisfying those needs. The coworkers became acquainted for the first time with the Nursing Process, its phases, care plans and the evaluation of the nursing interventions. The Nursing Process was practised as an experiment in six different departments and this experiment lasted for 3 weeks. The methods of the Nursing Process were presented in some textbooks and it was taught in the master's programme in nursing, but individualized care was not performed in any clinical setting at that time.

The major modernization of nursing care was started in the early 1990s, following the political changes in 1989. With the support of Dutch colleagues and the staff of the HOPE Project, the Charles University prepared the curriculum for a bachelor's programme in nursing. At the same time, seminars and workshops for nursing managers and university teachers were offered. These workshops covered both the philosophy of modern nursing and its practical implications for nursing care. When the bachelor's programme in nursing was launched in 1992, students were introduced to the theory of the Nursing Process. They practised using nursing documentation during their practical lessons at the health care facilities and their work followed the steps of Nursing Process. The practical lessons in each department were evaluated by means of a written nursing case study, which allowed the teacher to judge how well the student understood and used the Nursing Process.

After entering the workforce, these graduates with a bachelor's degree in nursing are usually entrusted with creating nursing documentation specific to a given department and helping other nurses to learn to use the Nursing Process. Nursing managers use their knowledge and skills to implement modern nursing. The basics of the Nursing Process have also been taught in the diploma programmes since 1995.

Endorsement

The Ministry of Health of the Czech Republic recommended the Nursing Process in 1998 as an appropriate way of providing nursing care. In a document called the 'Concept of Czech nursing', approved in 1998 by the Ministry of Health as the official strategy for the development of Czech nursing, the organization of nursing practice and nursing management is described in terms of the Nursing Process. According to this document the Nursing Process is the essential methodological framework for the implementation of the nursing objectives. The Nursing Process is a systematic and specific method of individualized approach to the nursing of every patient/client in the hospital or community setting, which is implemented in the following five integrated steps (Ministry of Health 1998: 9):

1. assessment of the patient;
2. definition of the nursing problems (diagnoses);
3. planning the individualized nursing care;
4. implementing the proposed care;
5. evaluating the effect of the care rendered.

Over and above this endorsement by the Ministry of Health, the nurse managers in some health care facilities motivate the nurses to use the Nursing Process.

Current status

According to the estimates of the faculty, Nursing Process documentation is being used in about 30% of hospital units, and individualized care is in place for about 8–10% of all hospitalized patients. There does not seem to be any outpatient health care facility where the Nursing Process is in use. There also does not seem to be any computerized hospital information system based on the Nursing Process. Some parts of nursing evaluation and intervention might be documented in this form, but it is not yet done comprehensively.

Both the nursing curriculum and the midwifery curriculum have been modernized, and the students are now well prepared to work according to modern nursing methods. There are modern Czech textbooks that are widely available. Some foreign textbooks have been translated as well.

There have been many textbooks (about 70–80 titles) published in the last 10 years. Some are written by Czech authors, some are translations. All of them describe or mention the Nursing Process in some way (Archalousova 2003: 99; Cervinková et al 2002: 75; Fendrychova 2000: 81, 2002: 145; Mastiliakova 2002: 187; Miksova et al 2002:143; Pacovsky 1994: 65; Ryslava 2002: 153; Stankova 1997: 193, 1999a: 66, 1999b: 48; Trachtova 1999: 186; Vasatkova et al 2002: 127).

The Nursing Process is not seen as a theory or a model in the Czech Republic, but as a methodology or an instrument. Teachers, therefore, use other nursing theories in combination with the Nursing Process. Without wanting to generalize, in the absence of empirical data, the faculty members regard Henderson, Gordon and Orem as popular theories in the country. The majority of teachers and schools also use the North American Nursing Diagnosis Association (NANDA) system of nursing diagnosis.

Nursing research is a new development in nursing in the Czech Republic. Although currently all nurses completing a bachelor's degree have to do a research project, there is no record of any research project on the Nursing Process as such.

CONCLUSION

The introduction of the Nursing Process into the Czech Republic is part of a range of changes that have happened over the last 20 years. So much has changed and is still changing, that little in-depth reflection has taken place about the individual aspects of the changes. The next 20 years will probably give nurses a better opportunity to reflect on their new systems, to research them and to make more informed decisions for themselves.

REFERENCES

Archalousova A 2003 Prehled vybranych osetrovatelskych modelu. Hradec Kralove, Nucleus

Cervinková E, Vorlickova H., Prikrylova L et al 2002 Osetrovatelske diagnozy. IDV PZ, Brno

Concept of Czech Nursing. Approved by the Ministry of Health as an official strategy of development of the Czech nursing 1998. Government Printers, Prague

Fendrychova J 2000 Osetrovatelske diagnozy v neonatologii. IDVPZ, Brno

Fendrychova J 2002 Osetrovatelske diagnozy v pediatrii. IDV PZ, Brno

Mastliakova D 2002 Uvod do osetrovatelstvi: systemovy pristup. Karolinum, Praha

Miksova Z, Fronkova M., Zajickova M et al 2002 Kapitoly z osetrovatelske pece. Nalios, Valasske Mezirici

Pacovsky V 1994 Osetrovatelska diagnostika. Karolinum, Praha

Ryslava M 2002 Osetrovatelské diagnozy a jejich prirazeni k vybranym lekarskym diagnozam v neonatologii. IDV PZ, Brno

Stankova M 1997 Zaklady teorie osetrovatelstvi. Karolinum, Praha

Stankova M 1999a Ceske osetrovatelstvi 4 – Jak provadet osetrovatelsky proces. IDV PZ, Brno

Stankova M 1999b Ceské osetrovatelstvi 3: Jak zavést ošetrovatelský proces do praxe. IDV PZ, Brno

Trachtova E 1999 Potreby nemocneho v osetrovatelskem procesu. IDV PZ, Brno

Vasatkova J et al 2002 Osetrovatelska dokumentace v nemocnici. IDV PZ, Brno

Chapter 12

The Nursing Process worldwide: what is its future?

Barbara Stevens Barnum

INTRODUCTION

Predicting the future of any process is an activity fraught with danger. Indeed, all one can hope is that the predictions are forgotten before the reality sets in. Nevertheless, my assignment is to look to the future of the Nursing Process, and I will try to do that. One thing is clear about the so-called Nursing Process: it has travelled around the world and has been widely adopted. In some cases, the adoption has been the choice of the nurses using it; in other cases, it has been thrust upon them by those in authority. The process has been hailed as necessary and helpful, and equally, it has been damned as a useless impediment. One thing is for certain: one must know the political/social history of the Nursing Process if we are to extrapolate its future.

One problem in assessing the future of the Nursing Process, particularly because it has spread worldwide, is that, despite this seeming universality, the process is better described by its radical disjuncture from one nation to another. The differences occur in the structure of the Nursing Process, in its application and, most importantly, in the cultural context.

Further, as author of this chapter, I can read and analyse the chapters presented in this book as background, but I cannot live the Nursing Process as applied in each country. Without a doubt, my assessment of the process will be primarily influenced by my own heritage, my immersion in the country where the Nursing Process originated. Unlike many authors in this book, for example, I cannot remember a time when the process was unknown to me.

Hence, I will never fully appreciate the impact that adopting the Nursing Process would have in a nation where it was a new concept. From the UK, Kelly (Chapter 2) makes an important point: that the Nursing Process played a part in switching the philosophy of nursing from a task-oriented one where there was little decision-making accountability to one where nursing moved toward greater intellectual autonomy. Others in this book have made similar observations. This function, obviously, is critical. Yet the Nursing Process was not such a turning point in the USA. It was not a signal in ending a task-orientated philosophy; which had already, in large part, happened.

With my own national 'blinders' on then, I shall attempt to discuss if not exactly a clear prediction of the process' future, at least some suggestions that might help us predict where it is likely to be heading. Wherever the Nursing Process appears, one cannot predict its future without understanding the structure, and the social and political history behind it. In the case of the Nursing Process, these elements interplay in ways that make it impossible to extract them from each other, so this paper weaves a complicated path from structure to politics and back again.

THE NURSING PROCESS: THE SCENE AT ITS EMERGENCE

Over its history, nursing has experimented with various forms of nursing theory. The strongest push for this activity came at the time when nursing was first attempting to prove itself to be of academic and scholarly worth (beginning in the late 1950s, but moving more strongly into the 1960s and early 1970s). In the attempts to move nursing into collegiate and university settings, a movement first seen on a large scale in the USA, nursing faculties attempted to follow the traditional pattern of occupations 'moving up'. Other would-be professions had found it essential to develop one or more theories of practice to underlie research, and so would nursing. It was seen as essential to copy the practices of the established professions.

Other professions used one of two patterns of theory development. Some professions worked within the confines of a single theory – chemistry and medicine, for example. If one were to study chemistry after years away from it, one would find that world very much changed. Valences, for example, have a different meaning now. But there would still be one basic theory of how the chemical world works, and it is used worldwide, even as it changes. Similarly, in modern times, medicine has always used a theory whereby things are explained in physiologic levels. The body is explained by its systems; the systems (e.g. the circulatory system) are explained by their organs; and the organs are explained by their cells. The pattern here has been little changed, albeit it has grown increasingly sophisticated. It is a system dominated by reductionism, where everything is explained by its smaller components, and the assumption is one of naïve realism, that is, the elements are perceived to exist independently of the observer/researcher.

Fields with only one theory usually do not discuss the theory much: it is simply accepted as 'how it is'. In these single-theory professions, growth is achieved by research that is in line with the standing theory.

Other fields develop multiple and competing theories. Psychology/psychiatry is an example of this sort. There are Freudians, Jungians, Adlerians, object relations devotees, behaviourists, schools of self-psychology, and many others. Each theory, when faced with the same case circumstances, interprets it differently according to the tenets of the particular theory. In these disciplines, discussion and development of theory is very important and, indeed, competitive.

Nursing is a discipline that has had multiple theories from the start of theory making (in the 1950s). Most of its theories bear the name of the theory's founder (e.g. Rogers, Orem, Roy, Levine, or Newman in the USA). Only two major theories fail to bear a founder's name, that is, the Problem Solving Method and the Nursing Process. Nevertheless, these are theories (or partial theories), albeit not always recognized as such. Although all these (and other) theories are still in use in the USA, most have almost been eclipsed by the Nursing Process.

Where theory and politics mix

The brief history given here relates what happened in the USA. Other countries that adopted the Nursing Process later had the advantage of skipping some of this early confusion. In the early era of professionalizing, schools of nursing were coping with an additional problem: how to teach 'everything'. The old nursing curricula were based on the medical model (body systems) and as new diseases and new therapies were discovered, the curriculum grew and grew. One of the faculty pressures was that of time. There was no criterion by which to glean down the growing body of content.

Additionally, there was a perceived need to differentiate the profession from other professions, especially from medicine. Part of 'growing up' as a profession was the need to have one's own theory, one's own independent practice. (Although I am focusing on a few selected aspects that were important in the thinking in the USA at this time, Traynor and Buus clarify in Chapter 3 other important themes of the era in their excellent analysis.)

At the time when these issues (a need for professionalizing and a need to control a runaway amount of programme content) held force, a critical study by Abdellah et al (1960) was published. The importance of this study was that it suggested new criteria, new subjects, by which nursing content could be ordered. In the USA, the shorthand for this new method was 'The 21 problems'. In actuality, the book suggested more than one approach, and these new organizational patterns suggested ways to make the expanding nursing content more manageable, more selective. This hallmark study totally changed the categories of nursing in the USA and it was based on research (a major goal in the profession's attempt to become scholarly).

Unfortunately, the document was also exploratory in nature, not surprising at this time. Depending on what portions of the book were selected as important, one could devise a Problem-based curriculum or a Nursing Process-based curriculum (albeit both of these forms were in their early states). Content could be varied also, ranging from patient problems, to nursing problems, to nursing goals. Commonly, faculty, who were attempting to follow these recipes for radical change, ended up, much as the authors had, throwing a little of everything into the pot, without recognizing that they were mixing and matching different formats.

For simplicity, the pure and unmixed structures of Problem-solving Nursing and Nursing Process are briefly explained here, simply because these two are still confused and intermixed. Problem-solving Nursing was an adaptation of a system then popular in non-nursing curricula. It was based on Dewey's (1938) formulation of rules for problem solving (i.e. the problematic method). Those procedures were the following.

1. Problem-solving starts with the recognition of an obstacle, situational or intellectual, a circumstance that interrupts the progress of the person's thought process or of his or her physical actions. At this stage, the obstacle is not clearly defined. It simply stops progress.
2. The person then attempts to clarify and define the problem. This involves much back and forth between the obstacle and the circumstances in which it occurs. Ultimately, the person defines the problem in a way that delimits and clarifies it. The wrong diagnosis here, obviously, will fatally flaw the rest of the process. For Dewey, problem definition was the most important part of problem-solving. Thereafter, the rest of the process tended to fall in line.
3. Alternate solutions suggest themselves once the problem has been defined. The problem solver reasons out solutions that seem to have the most hope of resolving the problem. Then he or she starts with the one most likely to make the problem go away. Notice, a goal is not superimposed here: the 'goal' is simply to get rid of the problem.

4. The problem solver tests the solution and, if it is not successful, the next potential solution is tested, and so forth until the problem is resolved. One will recognize here the familiar scientific process of hypothesis testing.

Notice that this process is not isolated to nursing. It could be problem-solving in cafeteria management, problem-solving for independent living or problem-solving in any domain at all. What made problem-solving a nursing theory was its linkage to nursing content. Problem-solving was the method; nursing provided the content.

The procedure given above sounds relatively simple; however, its application to nursing was not simple at all. Starting with the study by Abdellah et al (1960), some schools and institutions looked for *patient* problems (e.g. pain) and some looked for *nursing* problems (e.g. fluid and electrolyte imbalance). And when a problem was identified and solved, most institutions developed protocols of care so that the next time that 'problem' appeared, people would know what to do.

While this is a logical thing to do, most people failed to notice that this practice escaped the pure definition of problem solving, that is dealing with an indeterminate obstacle. Simply put, a solved problem was no longer a problem. Hence in nursing, the problematic form tended to be distorted from the start.

Nevertheless, problem-solving had a short run of popularity. The Weed (1978) problem-oriented system of charting was one example whereby nurses could only chart about a patient when they linked their notes to a definite problem. In some ways, problem-solving was a good match to nursing because nursing and nurses never lacked problems. The human environments for illness or well care were filled with problems that needed solutions.

Nevertheless, Problem-solving Nursing had a very short run in the USA because of a major change in the larger society: the advent and rapid development of the computer as a way of life and business. Historically, the computer changed the world with such rapidity that it amazed everyone. And when that happened, any system that was incompatible with 'computer thinking' got lost in the dusty trail. That included Problem-solving Nursing.

There were many difficulties with problem-solving methodology and computers. Chief among the difficulties is the fact that computers are not capable of handling subtleties or ambiguities. It would be impossible for a computer (without inputting hundreds or thousands of variables) to acknowledge that Nurse A and Nurse B might relate to the same patient successfully in two radically different ways. Computers give the same answers no matter who uses them; they are impervious to differences in the user. There is one right answer to every question for a computer, and the nursing situation is hardly ever that well defined.

Computers pushed first one nation, then the next, into accepting thought processes that were compatible with the functioning patterns of computers. This pattern is called systems thinking (or logistic thought). There was precedent for this form of thinking in the Abdellah et al (1960) book as well. What characterizes this pattern of thought is the following: the process is serial, with each step invariant and dependent on the findings at the prior step. And the steps and the findings at each step should be the same for anyone using the process.

One can easily recognize the Nursing Process in this description. First one assesses, then one plans, and so forth. No one is allowed to say, 'I don't feel like assessing right now. I think I'll intervene first, assess later'. Each step is dependent on what was found in the preceding step. The pattern is inflexible and prescribed.

As was the case in Problem-solving Nursing, the Nursing Process was a *nursing* procedure only because the process was applied to the content of nursing. One could just as easily have created the plumbing process. First the plumber *assesses* the situation (e.g. water is not going down the sink). Then he *diagnoses* the problem (e.g. clogged drain). Then he creates a *plan* (get out the snake), and then he *intervenes* (e.g. use the snake). Finally he *evaluates* (e.g. the water is running through the pipes again). In other words, the only thing that makes the Nursing Process *nursing* is that the process is applied to nursing content. The process is not unique to our profession.

One must also deal with the fact that people have many different versions of the Nursing Process, from the simplest, four steps, to some elaborations that go as far as seven or more steps. The familiar four-step includes: (1) assess the patient; (2) plan the care; (3) deliver the care; and (4) evaluate.

Plan, assess, implement and evaluate sounded good until people began to notice the logical gaps. First was the gap between assessment and planning. Obviously, the first did not lead directly to the second. One had to do something with the assessment data – and so came about nursing diagnosis, the first of many steps that would be added as the process evolved. Logically, one could derive at least the following steps: (1) patient assessment; (2) nursing diagnosis; (3) patient prognosis; (4) goal-setting; (5) therapeutic care planning; (6) care implementation; (7) evaluation of (a) patient status, (b) accuracy of prior assessment, (c) goal achievement, (d) accuracy of prognosis, (e) appropriateness of therapeutic choices, (f) effectiveness of care delivery, and (g) needed alterations in the plan (Barnum 1998).

Different places created different formulations of the Process. For example, the Ministry of Health of the Czech Republic recommended a five-step Nursing Process: (1) assess the patient; (2) define nursing problems (diagnoses); (3) plan individualized nursing care; (4) implement proposed care, and (5) evaluate effect of care rendered (Mellanová, Chapter 11). Uys of South Africa (Chapter 9) notes another formulation where five different steps involve (shortened and paraphrased): (1) identifying client's need; (2) identifying help that should be rendered; (3) intervention; (4) evaluation of results; and (5) recording of these steps.

Alas, when one applies logic to the Nursing Process, it becomes very involved, and a busy nurse taking care of patients may find it overwhelming. Hence, most nurses chose to ignore the logical gaps and go with the simpler formulations, letting their minds supply the missing pieces, usually without realizing they were doing it. Although many people squirm when different formulations (with different numbers of steps) are all called 'the Nursing Process', the truth is that they share more similarity than difference, namely their structure is logistic: (1) there is an invariant order to the steps;

(2) each step is dependent on the findings of the prior step; and (3) the system purports to be entirely independent of the user who is applying it.

The logistic structure fits the computer age. The Nursing Process had another advantage for a profession trying to prove that it was all grown up, namely the process *appeared* rational and infallible. All of this sounds good in 'computer speak', and it was sold to nursing in those terms. Alas, later research proved that the claims of rationality and infallibility were not always upheld. When actual testing was done, there was wide variance in responses. In fact, it is *not* the case that any two nurses using the system for a given patient come up with identical diagnoses and identical plans. The variance has always been an embarrassment to the advocates of the Nursing Process.

Development of the Nursing Process

In the USA, the development of the Nursing Process as a theory had a definite and predictable pattern. Research and adaptation simply began with the first step and sequentially went on from one step to the next. This meant that initial focus was on nursing assessment. In the USA, there was a great flurry as nurses learned how to do in-depth patient assessments, including history taking and, later, performance of physical examinations. Often this involved interactions with physicians who were the first teachers. Assessment techniques learned by nurses were identical to those taught to medical students.

When assessment had become a norm, it was predictable that the attention of nursing would turn to the next step, diagnosis, figuring out what conclusions could be drawn from the assessment data. Fortunately or unfortunately (and the opinion is divided), this movement occurred in an era when, as we saw earlier, nursing was striving to prove itself an independent profession. One of the thrusts, therefore, was to differentiate itself from medicine (even though some schools were still using physicians as teachers of patient assessment).

The politics of separatism carried the day in the USA, and thus began the movement of creating nursing diagnoses, a process to be eventually captured by the North American Nursing Diagnosis Association (NANDA). Although other early attempts at diagnostic categories were made, NANDA won the political battle hands down.

After diagnosis was well under way, it was predictable that nursing would come up with its own minimum information data set (Werley and Lang 1988). Aha, nursing could be computerized, taking out all the guesswork, or so went the theory. An effort to create protocol care plans associated with various diagnoses would be started next. Given the structure of the Nursing Process, and its ostensible separation from influence by the user, one can easily how this led to the formulation of care protocols. And where care could be put in the form of a protocol, it was, of course, ready for adaptation by information technology (see e.g. Ammenwerth, Chapter 5).

Then it followed that these nursing interventions would be formalized and categorized. The strongest thrust for this activity began and continued at the University of Iowa. Obviously, the question here was, what intervention 'fits' what diagnosis? And so it went – and will continue to go – through the rest of the Nursing Process. Evidence-based practice can be seen as the process intruding on the evaluation step. The fact that the Nursing Process ultimately extends into such validation processes is highly supportive of research. Hence, the process often became associated with the advancement and professionalizing of nursing (see Habermann, Chapter 7, for this effect in Germany).

How did it play in practice?

Never was a system of nursing more politicized than the Nursing Process. Advocates pushed the system until it was adopted worldwide by nations and health organizations as well. There was just one problem: nurses who actually had to work with the system were seldom happy. As we have seen throughout this book, acceptance was grudging in many cases. For example, Caribbean nurses reported great trouble with diagnoses (a la NANDA), awkward wording, legalistic terms, cultural misfits (Hewitt, Chapter 10). Even where the system became institutionalized, the acceptance was less than enthusiastic. As Taylor and Game (Chapter 8) report from Australia, the Nursing Process moved from: 'Ah, yeah, it's more of American bunkum . . .' to begrudging acceptance. From Finland, we find Välimäki and Kaunonen (Chapter 6) noting that only parts of the Nursing Process seemed to be put into practice. Uys of South Africa (Chapter 9) notes that many nurses had difficulty applying the process and that the requisite documentation was very difficult. Ward (Chapter 4), gives an interesting example of how the Nursing Process came into play when a new turf (community mental health) was being carved out for relatively independent nursing practice.

THE FUTURE OF THE NURSING PROCESS: MODELS OF THE FUTURE

In the history of nursing, as is true of any movement in a society at large, each system (in this case, the organizing of nursing care) finds the method by which it organizes periodically replaced by another method. This happens when the irritants of the reigning method become too burdensome. Every method has its downside; there is no such thing as a perfect schema. The downside of a given method may show up sooner, if the environment for which it was designed changes. For example, a system that focuses on quality may be too costly in an era focusing on economic stringency. Or a system that focuses on the individuality of patients may yield to a social system focused on group behaviours and goals.

Whatever the downside of the reigning method, it is a certainty that the new method will be one that solves the immediate problems of the old system. Hence, we have a continual process: a reigning method, the method's flaws emerge, a new method without these flaws replaces the old method, the new method's flaws eventually become apparent, then yet another method is initiated, and the process continues. Since a new method may retain some of the better elements of the old method, one could view this process as an eternal dialectic.

If we look at the flaws of the Nursing Process, they will give us a clue as to the nature of the method that will replace it. Notice, if there was any doubt, this presumes (on my part) that the Nursing Process is not eternal. The question is not whether it will be replaced, but when and why. In the chapters of this book, we saw several flaws in the Nursing Process. First, the system, gathering strength as a political movement, was often crammed down people's throats. Whether this was a matter of re-educating people to a better way or simply a sign of the system's power to be a top gun is a matter of one's interpretation.

The system was advanced and enforced by the powerful. Usually that involved education versus practice (academics over practitioners) – with educators the ones forcing the theory into both education (curricula) and practice. This, then, set the stage for a major division in nursing – a 'we versus they' mentality. In many cases, the Nursing Process was a useful tool for educating students, but what about practice?

What can we infer from the nationwide comments we read in this book concerning Nursing Process as it applies in practice? Here we have a system that was greeted with lukewarm enthusiasm at best – and more typically, with resistance. Is it possible that everyone in practice was wrong? Or is the Nursing Process a system that simply was not meeting the needs of the practitioners? Logic dictates that all these practising nurses cannot be entirely wrong.

One cause for resistance in the practice arena was that the system apparently added complexity. Complexity may have been reflected in the nurses being forced to use intellectual patterns that seemed less relevant than the prior patterns. Complexity also was reflected in increased care work and increased paperwork. Many times the system was seen as adding a burden to nursing, not as assisting it.

How was Nursing Process welcomed? By others? Seldom. The process was often met by medicine with mockery. How was it accepted by nurses? Leadership, especially academics could rightly be accused of forcing the process on the practice environment. Did the 'forcing' achieve what was envisioned by the leadership? In some measure, yes, but often not at all.

Consider that insanity reported in the Caribbean article (Hewitt, Chapter 10) in which the Process was accepted by academe and the official Nursing Council of Jamaica, and was included in the Caribbean Standards of Nursing Care but not applied much in practice. One telling note of problems of cultural context in translation is the following. Although the Ministry of Health approved the recommendations (including the Nursing Process), there was insufficient paper to meet the documentation required by the system. Here we are talking about the insanity of attempting to enforce a system without appropriate resources.

In short, we have a system that has developed from a logical plan but one that does not 'fit' the work environment in many cultures, except with distortion, and distortion that may cause additional work (real work or documentation work) without additional payoff in care benefits. Consider the criterion of utility: if a system has been in existence over 25 years and is still more characterized by poor implementation than good, this must speak of flaws in the system. Remember, earlier we addressed another structural problem: the fact that the process did not deliver on the uniformity of practice it promised.

Recall in the preceding discussion we were searching for the *flaws* in the Nursing Process so as to predict its replacement. (We will come back to this.) This does not mean that the system was without merit. Indeed, it strove to correct the flaws in the preceding systems. One major flaw of the preceding systems in many nations was that they did not encourage an intellectual or systemized approach to the field. Certainly these older formulations did not pattern themselves on thought processes that would be acceptable in a collegiate setting.

Did the Nursing Process serve an important function in the era of striving to make nursing professional and respected? Yes. Many of our authors spoke to the utility of the Nursing Process in the academic setting (see e.g. Välimäki and Kaunonen of Finland, Chapter 6). Some stressed that it created a different mentality from the past focus on tasks. Uys from South Africa (Chapter 9) noted that it served to make nurses conscious of nursing elements that had not been consciously considered earlier. Did the Nursing Process enable nursing to build a competitive model that separated it from medicine? Yes, it did that by developing nursing's own language, particularly in diagnostic categories. In the march of history, the Nursing Process adequately managed many flaws of the prior systems.

But do advantages of the process hold into the present time? The answer is simple: its flaws are showing. A clear and present flaw is one of environmental changes that have occurred since the system was put in place (albeit its implementation was often partial). Managed care has grown worldwide, and this has demanded a focus on economy and efficiency. Yet here we have a method, the Nursing Process, which is known for its extensive use of resources, especially nursing hours.

Further, and more important, the era of managed care demands a cooperating, not a competing model among and between professions. And the Nursing Process has been specifically designed as a competitive model.

Moreover, the model may be incompatible with new forms of nursing practice, namely nurse practitioner roles (new in the USA, more mature in some other locations, and yet to be formulated in others). However, the nurse practitioner role demands a tight interface with medicine, where 'speaking the same language' is essential.

It seems to me that we are sitting on the cusp, waiting to see what method will next rear its head and challenge the Nursing Process. It is impossible to say what model will emerge, but it might be a model using operational thought – a system made popular in medicine by the procedure of differential diagnosis. The last nursing major theory to use operational thought was Orem's, and one of its advantages was that nurses, students and practitioners liked it. Obviously, the content might be different in a new method, but the structure of the thinking would be similar. The operational thought pattern uses 'either or' reasoning (e.g. either it is benign or malignant). If malignant, either it is operable or treatable by other means. If by other means, . . . and so forth.

The operational model would provide the following characteristics: (1) compatible with the medical model and collegial in nature; (2) compatible with branching logic in computer-driven systems, which will still be around; and (3) more streamlined than the Nursing Process system (i.e. designed for economy and efficiency, not for generating more work). Such a differential diagnosis model (using operational thought processes) and possibly shared with medicine, is only one possibility. Of course, if I had to bet, this would be my choice.

In the USA, we also find a unique growing counterculture that challenges the systems model represented by the Nursing Process. The model is that of holistic nursing. Although the term, holism, has sometimes been applied to the Nursing Process, that is a misnomer. *Holism*, when used with Nursing Process, can only mean that all the pieces have been collected, that the care is 'whole' in the sense of everything being done. The Nursing Process is a method of steps, of pieces, *not* a method of holism. Doing 'everything' does not mean one has approached the task holistically.

In the USA today, we do not really have nursing so much as two nursings – that based on a scientific model (including use of the Nursing Process), and that based on a holistic view of the indivisible human being, in which he or she cannot be divided into components or component processes, such as happens in the Nursing Process.

Take, for example, holistic principle of 'being with' the patient put forward by Dossey and colleagues (2000). 'Being with' therapies, she notes, do not involve 'doing' for the patient; they involve benefits derived from the simple presence of the nurse. Obviously, theories of holistic nursing are far more complex than this one illustration but they arise from a different philosophy than the one behind the Nursing Process. The different philosophies lead to different conclusions about patients, different conclusions about what nurses should do and different conclusions about how care should be evaluated. Will both types of nursing continue to exist side by side? Will they come to respect each other, as opposed to the present competition? Will one side 'win' over the other, asserting its protocols of care? Will this format of holistic nursing take root in other nations? Clearly, this is another way in which the Nursing Process might be replaced, albeit a less likely one.

Alternately, a new system not yet emerged may replace the Nursing Process and, if so, we will simply have to wait until it appears on the horizon. Fortunately, my task was not to describe the replacement waiting in the wings, but simply to pronounce on the future of the Nursing Process. In one sense, this makes my job easy because no process lasts forever. The question then becomes, how long will the Nursing Process be around before it is replaced? And the answer is: until something better comes along. Given the irritants in the process, one can be sure that people are struggling to create that alternative, even as we speak.

REFERENCES

Abdellah F G, Beland I L, Martin A, Matheney R V 1960 Patient-centered approaches to nursing. Macmillan Company, New York

Barnum B 1998 Nursing theory: analysis, application, evaluation. Lippincott, Philadelphia

Dewey J 1938 Logic: the theory of inquiry. Henry Holt, New York

Dossey B M, Keegan L, Guzzetta C E 2000 Holistic nursing: A handbook for practice, 3rd edn. Aspen, Gaithersburg, MD

Weed L 1978 Medical records, medical education, and patient care. Case Western Reserve University, Cleveland

Werley H H, Lang N M (eds) 1988 Identification of the nursing minimum data set. Springer, New York

Index